13 Secrets to Optimal Aging

How Bio-Identical Hormone Therapy Can Help You Achieve a Better Quality of Life and Longevity

Dr. Kelly Miller, DC, NMD, FASA, FBAARM, CFMP

13 Secrets to Optimal Aging: How Bio-Identical Hormone Therapy Can Help You Achieve a Better Quality of Life and Longevity

Book 1 of the *Health Restoration Series*
      Series Editor, George Ann Gregory, Ph.D.

Printed by CreateSpace, An Amazon.com Company
CreateSpace, Charleston, SC

ISBN-13: 978-0-9979113-0-5
ISBN-10: 0997911301

Table of Contents

Foreword

Notes

Medical care in the U.S. is in trouble, big trouble. We spend far more on health care than any other country. We take more prescription drugs than any other people on the planet. What do we get for having the most expensive health care and for taking the most drugs? When compared to every other major Western country, we have a shorter life span and more chronic illnesses. In fact, on nearly every health indicator we finish dead last or next to last.

Clearly what we are doing is not working. We need a better path.

Dr. Kelly Miller's book, *13 Secrets to Optimal Aging: How Bio-Identical Hormone Therapy Can Help You Achieve A Better Quality Of Life And Longevity* provides such a path to get us out of the mess we are in.

I was trained as a conventional family practitioner. When I began practicing what I was taught, I quickly realized something was terribly wrong. I found myself treating my patients with too many drugs that were not treating the underlying cause of their illness and then having to use other drugs to treat the side effects from the first drug used. Most importantly, I realized my patients were not getting better, nor were they going to get better with the therapies I had available. I quickly realized that I could not, in good conscience, practice medicine this way for the next forty years. *Problem*

With the help of a patient, I began researching the use of natural items in order to provide the body with the optimal level of nutrients that allow it not only to heal from injury, but also to maintain optimal health. *Note V: Very import*

One of the first items I started using was a bio-identical, natural hormone. My father was my first patient treated. A combination of bio-identical, natural testosterone and natural thyroid hormone had a dramatic positive effect on his health. Once I saw the changes in my father, I knew that was the type of medicine I wanted to practice. Now, twenty-one years later, I still find medicine interesting and I still research and use natural therapies.

Dr. Miller has written a much-needed book that explains the theory and practice of how to incorporate the use of bio-identical, natural hormones in order to treat illness and to help maintain optimal health. He also explains, in an easy-to-read format the proper tests to order in order to evaluate the hormonal system. Dr. Miller also provides case histories that further help the reader understand the importance of balancing the hormonal system with bio-identical, natural hormones.

"Every patient that I see gets a hormonal and nutritional evaluation. I have witnessed countless patients improve their health by using bio-identical, natural hormones in order to provide the body with the raw materials it needs to optimally function.

Dr. Miller's book is a must-read for those seeking a healthy approach. My colleagues would do well to read this book and learn about how important it is to have a balanced hormonal system. I highly recommend this book for all interested in natural healing methods.

David Brownstein, M.D.

Author of 13 books including *Overcoming Thyroid Disorders and Iodine: Why You Need It, Why You Can't Live Without It.*

www.drbrownstein.com

Preface

This book is designed to educate those who are curious about hormone therapy, who want to know how to use hormone therapy safely, and who want to maximize their results for optimal aging. It is also designed to educate the reader about the hormones in the body, the many functions they perform, and how they work together. In my clinical experience of over thirty-five years of helping over 15,000 patients, I have found there are four basic concerns middle-aged and elderly people share about the aging process. I hate to even use terms like middle-aged and elderly, as I have just turned age sixty and don't feel like either of these.

The first concern many people have about aging is that they are afraid they won't retain their mental faculties. Many of my friends and patients have had to take care of spouses or parents who suffered from dementia or Alzheimer's disease. They do not want to wind up that way, and there is no reason they should have to. As you will soon learn, many of the hormones that are discussed in this book are involved in the function of memory and recall.

The second concern many people have about aging is that they will lose the ability to ambulate on their own. Loss of mobility in the aging population is caused by several factors, including arthritic dysfunctional joints (spine, hips, knees, and feet), strokes or heart attacks, fractures from falls, balance problems, neuropathy, or generalized deconditioning following an extended hospitalization. The sex hormones are naturally anti-inflammatory, encourage muscle and bone strength and health, and enhance and maintain neurological, cardiovascular, and immune health.

The third concern many people have about aging is a loss of libido or sexual function. Half of divorces of middle-aged couples in the U.S. today are probably related to sexual disinterest or dysfunction. Libido, the desire for sex, is natural and a reflection of a healthy status of an individual. The information in this book will help both men and women have a better understanding of why erectile dysfunction occurs in men and why women become disinterested or experience painful sex. The good news for both men and women is that these problems can almost always be resolved without medication and without unpleasant or dangerous side effects.

The fourth concern many people have as they age is that they will become unattractive to their spouse or the opposite sex—that no one will find them attractive any more. They worry they will be too fat, too saggy, too wrinkly, or the like. As you will learn, the hormones help maintain muscle tone and mass, bone strength, reduce fat and wrinkles, and moisturize the tissues. Supplementing bio-identical hormones in a balanced manner has a positive effect on muscles, bones, heart, and skin, even the face.

There are several important concepts that are presented in this book. One important fact that many are not aware of is that most of the hormones in the body are derived from cholesterol. Most of us have been inappropriately conditioned to think that the lower an individual's cholesterol is the better. This is just not true. Adequate cholesterol levels are essential to having optimal hormone production. The second fact is that there is vast difference between synthetic hormones and bio-identical hormones, and it is the synthetic hormones, not the bio-identical hormones, that are associated with increased risk for heart attacks, strokes, blood clots, and some cancers. The third fact is that there are multiple ways to test and administer the hormones. If you are already on a hormone replacement therapy, you might want to re-consider the methodology you are currently using.

The next important concept to understand is that only *physiological* doses of bio-identical hormones should be used. This means that an individual should not be taking a higher level of hormones than a younger, healthy version of themselves could produce on their own. Dosing of hormones should be individualized, based on the genetic, bio-chemical, and physical attributes of each person. Another important concept to appreciate is that a single hormone deficiency *never* exists. Because of the complex interrelationship of the endocrine system and cascading of the sex hormones, having a single hormone deficiency is impossible. Each hormone has both *synergistic* and *antagonistic* hormones that are influenced by a deficiency in that hormone.

Another important aspect of understanding sex hormones is that the measurement of the levels of hormones only represents half the equation in optimal hormone function. The other equally important aspect of the equation is *receptor sensitivity*. Even if the hormone level appears optimum, if there is not appropriate receptor sensitivity the individual will have deficiency symptoms because the hormone is unable to bind to the receptor, resulting in the cell being

x

unable to use the hormone. Actually, the more receptors tissues or an organ has for a particular hormone the more important that particular hormone is to the function of those tissues or organ. A hormone deficiency/imbalance produces dysfunction first in those tissues or organ having the greatest number of cell receptors. An example of this is the one hundred percent increased risk for a heart attack in men when their testosterone levels have become reduced by half of what their levels were when they were age twenty-five because of the tremendous amount of testosterone receptors in the heart. Ultimately, hormone levels reflect, in many ways, the relative health or health potential. Low levels of hormones are the reflection of the cumulative effects of genetic variances and emotional, mechanical, nutritional, and environmental stressors on the body. The levels are a scorecard of how well an individual is doing in the aging process: Is the individual doing average, above average, or below average?

Supplementing hormones helps to improve body functions immediately and dramatically, but consideration should be made to what are the cause or causes for any hormone depletion. For example, advertisements ask men do you have low T (testosterone). The next question—if the answer is a yes—should be why do you have low testosterone. Is it because of emotional stress, or is it because of insulin and blood sugar dysregulation, for example? While supplementing with testosterone may help, the causes, such as emotional stress, must be eliminated or the insulin/blood sugar dysregulation corrected. Eliminating the cause results in rising testosterone levels, and the need for supplementation is reduced. A similar approach should be taken in analyzing the most common problem aging women have with low progesterone levels. Consideration should be given as to what is causing the deficiency.

Every month, one million people in the world turn age sixty-five. In the U.S., the average sixty-five-year-old American is on six to ten prescription medications. The United States of America constitutes only five percent of the world's population, yet accounts for fifty percent of the consumption of prescription medications worldwide. Additionally, the United States ranks first in cancer and cardiovascular disease in the world.

While people in the U.S. have been living longer than people did one hundred years ago, they have not been living well as they age. Even though the U.S. prides itself in what an advanced health care system it has, the British, the Greeks, and the Japanese have higher rates of longevity with less debilitating disease as they age than people in the U.S. For the first time in fifty plus years, predicted longevity rates have decreased for American children. The average American who doesn't die of a heart attack or metastatic cancer much too often spends their last months or years in a nursing home, in a diaper, unable to ambulate on their own, and unable to recollect the people they love and the events that shaped their lives.

This book is part of the remedy to avoid such an existence. This book is about the pursuit and realization of a higher quality of life and a longer healthier life. The thirteen secrets contained in this book are your hormones. Natural bio-identical hormones are not the complete solution for perfect health, but they are powerful tools to enhance optimal aging. You must still eat wholesome foods, drink pure water, get regular quality sleep, get regular exercise, breathe fresh clean air, and renew your mind with positive thoughts. However, there is no doubt that this approach adds many quality years to life. This information is life changing and life saving. I wish you the best in your pursuit of health and happiness.

Kelly Miller, DC, NMD, FASA, FBAARM, CFMP

Acknowledgements

I could not have written this book without the support and encouragement of my best friend and soul mate, Dr. Debra Hoffman. She is the best person I have ever known. I would also like to thank my mentor, Dr. Paul Tai, for his patient and enthusiastic teachings in Aging and Regenerative Medicine. I give thanks to my sister, Dr. George Ann Gregory, for her editing and my brother, Bruce Miller, and my long-time patient, Teresa Ellis, for googling data for me. Thank you to Jennifer Brown for her transcription, Deepali Gupta for her illustrations, and Emz Wright for the book cover.

I have been guided by the following Biblical passages.

Proverbs 8:1-36, 9:1

Does wisdom not cry out, and understand lift up her voice? She takes her stand on the top of the high hill, beside the way, where the paths meet. She cries out by the gates, at the entry of the city, at the entrance of the doors: "To you, O men, I call, and my voice is to the sons of men. O you simple ones, understand prudence, and you fools, be of understanding heart. Listen, for I will speak of excellent things, and from the opening of my lips, will come right things. For my mouth will speak truth: wickedness is an abomination to my lips. All the words of my mouth are with righteousness; nothing crooked or perverse is in them. They are all plain to him that understands, and right to those who find knowledge. Receive my instruction, and not silver, and knowledge rather than choice gold; For wisdom is better than rubies, and all the things one may desire cannot be compared to her. "I, wisdom, dwell with prudence, and find out knowledge and discretion. The fear of the Lord is to hate evil; pride and arrogance and the evil way and perverse mouth I hate. Counsel is mine, and sound wisdom; I am understanding, I have strength. By me kings reign, and rulers decree justice. By me princes rule, and nobles, all the judges of the earth. I love those who love me, and those who seek me diligently will find me. Riches and honor are with me, enduring riches and righteousness. My fruit is better than gold, yes, than fine gold, and my revenue than fine silver. I transverse the way of righteousness, in the midst of justice, That I may cause those who love me to inherit wealth, that I may fill their treasures. "The Lord possessed me, at the beginning of His way, before His works of old. I have been established from everlasting. From the beginning, before there was an earth. When there were no depths I was brought forth, when there were no fountains abounding with water. Before the mountains were settled, before the hills, I was brought forth; while as yet He had not made the earth or the fields, or the primal dust of the world. When He prepared the heavens, I was there, when He drew a circle on the face of the deep, When He established clouds above, when He strengthened the fountains of the deep, When He assigned to the sea its limit, so that the waters would not transgress His command, when He marked out the foundations of the earth, Then I was beside Him as a master craftsman; and I was daily His delight, rejoicing always before Him, Rejoicing in His inhabited world, and my delight was with the sons of men. "Now therefore, listen to me my children, for blessed are those who keep my ways. Hear instruction and be wise, and do not disdain it. Blessed is the man who listens to me, watching daily at my gates, waiting at the posts of my doors. For whoever finds me finds life, and obtains favor from the Lord; But he who sins against me wrongs his own soul; all those who hate me love death." Wisdom has built her house, she has hewn out her seven pillars. *NKJV*

Proverbs 9:9-11

Give instruction to a wise man, he will be yet wiser: teach a just man, and he will increase in learning. For the fear of the Lord is the beginning of wisdom; and the knowledge of the holy is understanding. For by me thy days shall be multiplied and the years of thy life shall be increased. *NKJV*

James: 13-17

Who is wise and understanding among you? Let him show by good conduct that his works are done in the meekness of wisdom. But if you have bitter envy and self-seeking in your hearts, do not trust and lie against the truth. This wisdom does not descend from above, but is earthly, sensual, demonic. For where envy and self-seeking exist, confusion and every evil thing are there. But the wisdom that is from above is first pure, then peaceable, gentle, willing to yield, full of mercy and good fruits, without partiality and without hypocrisy. *NKJV*

Disclaimer

This publication is designed to provide scientific, authoritative, and personal anecdotal information in regard to the subject matter covered. The reader understands that the author is not engaged in rendering professional services. If you require medical, psychological, or any other expert assistance, please seek the services of a professional.

The information, personal experiences, anecdotal stories, procedures, and suggestions contained in the book are not intended to replace the services of a trained health-care professional or to serve as a replacement for a health-care professional's advice and care. You should consult a health-care professional regarding any of this information, ideas, personal experiences, anecdotal stories, procedures, supplements, drug therapies, or any other information from this book.

The author hereby specifically disclaims any and all liability arising directly or indirectly from the use or application of any of the products, ideas, procedures, drug therapies, or suggestions contained in this book and any errors, omissions, and inaccuracies in the information contained herein. The treatments and supplements included in this book are for identification purposes only and are not intended to recommend or endorse the product.

Warning

This book is intended for readers and physicians to evaluate hormone deficiencies that occur in the human body. However, it is not intended for pregnant women or nursing women, nor is it intended for individuals under the age of 18.

Optimum and deficient values presented within this book do not necessarily correspond to the reference values found in local laboratories. The values and references used in this book are purely subjective and come from the author's own personal experiences and by other physicians who have shared their experiences.

The reader should not base his or her assessment solely on the values given in this book. Laboratories determine hormonal imbalances, and health-care professionals determine correct approaches.

Laboratory values within this book constitute only some of the information the reader should gather. Additional emphasis should be placed on clinical evaluation, signs, and symptoms. Many other clinical and laboratory tests should be used before deciding on a diagnosis and/or treatment. A reader should always seek a physician's advice before deciding to institute any form of medical treatment.

Chapter 1: Why You Should Consider Bio-Identical Hormone Therapy

There are three major reasons why you should consider bio-identical hormone therapy, and all three have to do with the quality of life as you age. Generally speaking, as we age, our hormone levels decline. Specific hormones begin to decline at different ages. For example, *testosterone* and *DHEA* begin to decline at about age twenty-five, and *progesterone* at about age thirty-five. The age and rate of decline can vary from individual to individual due to genetics, trauma, environmental toxins, and the six essentials to health: what we eat, what we drink, how we rest, how we exercise, what/how we breathe, and what we think.[1]

There has been a general decline in testosterone levels in American men over the last three decades as documented by the Massachusetts Male Aging Study, a large on-going epidemiological research project involving tens of thousands of participants.[2] Almost ninety percent of American women suffer from PMS. (Pre-Menstrual Symptoms), caused by a relative imbalance of estrogen to progesterone.[3] Hormone levels are often a reflection of the various emotional, mechanical, and chemical stressors on the body. There is abundant evidence indicating that, especially in the U.S., the average individual is over-burdened with food additives like *MSG* (mono-sodium glutamate), and a*spartame* (Nutrasweet[T]), high fructose corn syrup (*HFCS*), and *trans-fats*. In addition, there is exposure from heavy metals like mercury and lead, *PBA*s in plastics, *PCB*s in ocean fish and butter, and chlorinated pesticides in the food chain.[4] All of these play havoc with the endocrine (hormone) system.

They are *endocrine disrupters*. Specifically, both HFCS and trans-fat have an inhibitory effect on the hypothalamic receptor sites accepting *leptin.*[5] Leptin is a master hormone produced from our fat cells that signal the satiety center in the hypothalamus that we are full. Without this signal, we overeat, causing overweight/obesity and *insulin resistance*. This, in turn, decreases tissue-building hormones like DHEA and testosterone. Increased body fat increases estrogen, which slows *thyroid* hormone function. Many environmental toxins cause hypothalamus/*pituitary* dysregulation. These glands function to monitor and signal the adrenals, gonads, and thyroid to produce different hormones. Some of the these environmental chemicals that mimic estrogen cause endocrine (hormone) disruption. These toxins can also contribute to *receptor resistance*, which has the same net result in the body as lowered hormone levels do.

All of the cells in the body have many receptor sites for hormones and chemicals that include Vitamin D, *adrenaline, cortisol* and thyroid hormone as well as other hormones. The more receptor sites on the membrane of the cells of a specific organ the more dependent that specific organ is on the hormone. For example, a woman's vagina has an abundance of estrogen receptors. When estrogen levels reduce to a certain level in the aging process, the tissue dries and shrinks due to lack of receptor stimulation from the estrogen.

Another important factor in maintaining healthy hormone levels is the interrelationship among vitamins, minerals, and anti-oxidants. This is why what we eat, or don't eat, has such a profound influence on hormones. Vitamins, minerals, and anti-oxidants are absolutely essential for five functions related to hormones— providing nutrients for (1) the tissues that make the hormones, (2) the enzymes involved in the conversion process of one hormone to another, (3) the enzymes involved in detoxification of the hormones, (4) the organs involved in hormone detoxification, and (5) the mitochondrial energy for the organs that both produce the hormones and detoxify them. Ensuring adequate nutritional intake of all these co-factors equates to better hormone production and cell membrane receptor sensitivity.

Optimum nutritional intake helps to maintain hormones at higher and longer levels. Even with this optimal nutritional intake, at some point, bio-identical hormone therapy needs to be initiated to maximize quality longevity and preserve more youthful levels of hormones. When centenarians have been evaluated, it has been found that key nutrients like Vitamin D, Vitamin C, B Vitamins, zinc, selenium, and magnesium are higher than the average person forty years younger. Likewise, when these centenarian's hormone levels were analyzed, their DHEA and *melatonin* levels are higher than many sixty-year-olds.[3]

When aging individuals supplement with bio-identical hormones in a balanced manner, the cells in all parts of the body, including the brain, bone, muscles, heart, blood vessels, digestive system, skin, respond in a more youthful manner. Hormones make protein, and proteins make all our cells—muscles, bones, and skin.

2

As hormone levels decline in the aging process, the body literally shrinks and dries up. Our mouth, lips, and eyes are less moist. Our skin is dryer. Our organs become stiffer, drier, and smaller. Everything shrinks—our muscles, bones, and bladders—even our sex organs. Hormones moisturize and regenerate the muscles, bones, mouth, eyes, and skin. With hormones, the skin thickens and becomes softer. The mouth produces more saliva. The eyes produce more tears. There is less dry mouth and dry eyes. Even the vaginal tissue thickens and become moist again so that sexual intercourse is no longer painful.

After *bio-identical* hormone therapy, I have, time and time again, observed and heard reports from my patients that their memory and recall have improved, their muscle tone and size have improved, their body/visceral fat has reduced, their cardiovascular, digestive, and immune function have improved, their skin and hair have improved, their sexual function has improved, and their sleep, energy and endurance have improved.

The bio-identical hormone therapy allows us to prolong our creative and productive years. *The Outliers* by Malcolm Gladwell—a book I enjoyed reading—discusses the concept that it takes ten thousand hours of focused practice to become world-class at anything: a sport, a vocation, or an art.[6] There are only a very few of us who achieve this at an early age. This achievement is seen in Olympic teenage gymnasts. Bobby Fischer is also an example of a person who became a world-class chess champion at a young age. While each of us has unique qualities and abilities, for many of us we don't figure out what we are really good at and enjoy doing until middle age, however. Sometimes, it is not until a second, or even a third career, that we develop the passion and skill-set to become world-class at something. I have many friends and business colleagues who fall into this category. I am attracted to people who have an enthusiasm and passion for life. I often ask my friends and my patients who are middle-aged, "What could you accomplish if you had another forty to fifty years of quality life?"

Many Americans look forward to their retirement to have the time to do the things they always wanted to do. Unfortunately, too many Americans have health issues that prevent their plans for the *golden years* from ever occurring. Aging should be and can be a blessing. The goal is to age like a fine wine. Gray hair is a glorious crown. Aging is about acquiring wisdom and passing it on. It is good to stop, appreciate, and smell the roses of life. Life, like your hormones is about balance. Do you have a strategy for quality longevity? If you want to live long and feel good, you need a game plan. You need a strategy to achieve that goal. The information contained in this book is part of my plan and part of the plan of many of many patients to achieve optimal aging.

The *13 secrets* that will allow you to achieve optimal aging are maintaining optimal levels of (1) cholesterol, which is the *source* of all the sex hormones and vitamin D, (2) *pregnenolone*, the *mother* of all the sex hormones, (3) DHEA, the father of all the sex hormones, (4) progesterone, (5) cortisol, (6) aldosterone, (7) testosterone, (8) estrogen, (9) growth hormone, (10) melatonin, (11) vitamin D, and keeping your (12) thyroid and (13) adrenals functioning optimally. If you are reading this book, it is probably because you either have a specific complaint, illness, or disease you are searching an answer for, or because you are investigating the possibilities that aging and regenerative medicine has to offer. Bio-identical hormone therapy could be part of the solution you are looking for. The remaining chapters provide you information about what I feel is the safest and optimum application of this technology.

Chapter 1 References

1. Morter MT Jr, *Your Health, Your Choice,* Frederick Fell Publishers, 2012.
2. O'Donell AB, Araujo AB, McKinley JB. The health of normally aging men. The Massachusetts Male Aging Study (1987-2004). *Exp. Geronitol. July; 39(7);975-84.*
3. Tai PL, *8 Powerful Secrets to Anti-Aging,* Health Secrets, USA, 2005, Dearborn, Michigan.
4. Blaylock RL, *Excitotoxins: The Taste That Kills*, Health Press, Sante Fe, New Mexico.
5. Tai PL, *The Thin Factors: A Super Weight Loss Program!,* Health Secrets, USA, Dearborn, Michigan.
6. Gladwell M, *Outliers: The Story of Success,* Amazon.com/books , 2011.

Chapter 2: How Our Hormone Systems Work ✓

Our hormones are controlled by what is called *negative feedback,* which is a reaction that causes an increase or decrease in function. Here is how it works. The hypothalamus is a gland near the center of the brain. It is responsible for monitoring all internal sensory data in the body. It constantly monitors the amount of any hormone circulating in the blood. It is similar to a thermostat, but instead of monitoring a specific temperature, it monitors a specific hormone level. If hormone levels fall below a certain level, the hypothalamus secretes a *releasing hormone* that signals the pituitary gland to produce a *stimulating hormone* that travels to the *target organ* that causes the target organ to produce the necessary hormone. Primarily, these target organs are the thyroid, adrenals, and gonads. This is covered in more detail on the discussion of each specific hormone later in this book.

At the other end of the spectrum, when the hypothalamus senses the hormone levels have risen sufficiently, it stops producing the releasing hormone that signals the pituitary to produce the stimulating hormone that communicates to the target gland. The hormone production stops for a while. This happens 24/7, in two-to-three hour cyclic patterns. For instance, testosterone and cortisol levels should always be highest in the morning. These levels fluctuate every two to three hours. Consequently, there is a constant roller coaster-like pattern of hormone production in a twenty-four hour cycle. Production of the hormones is the first half of the story of hormones.

The second half of the story takes place at the receptor sites in the cells of the different tissues of the body. The more receptor sites for a specific hormone located in a particular organ the more dependent that organ is on the specific hormone to function optimally. For example, the heart has more testosterone receptor sites than any other organ in the body other than the testes. What this tells us is that heart function is testosterone dependent to a certain extent. Because of this, when a man loses 50 percent of his testosterone levels, his risk for heart attack doubles, independent of any other factors. [1] Does this mean people who have lower levels of testosterone are at increased risk for a heart attack? *Absolutely!* However, as I said, the first half of the story is about hormone production. The second half of the story is the function of the receptors.

It is not enough simply to have the hormone at a certain level. The hormone must bond with the receptor to enhance cellular function. Most of us have heard of insulin resistance, for example. Insulin resistance occurs even when there is adequate, even many times elevated, levels of insulin being produced, but the receptor sites have become resistant to binding with the insulin. The receptors are no longer receptive to the messenger, which is the hormone. The receptor becomes like your thirteen-year-old son or daughter. They aren't listening to your message anymore. They are tuning you out.

Another common example of this is when all hormone levels for the thyroid are within reference range in the blood chemistry panels, yet the patient has all the classic symptoms of hypothyroidism. The *TSH* (*thyroid stimulating hormone*) produced in the pituitary appears normal. The free *T3* (*triiodothyronine*) and *T4* (*thyroxine*) levels appear to be normal, which means adequate reference range thyroid hormones are being produced and converted. The *TPO* (*thyroid peroxidase*) level is within reference range. This means there is no antibody being produced against the thyroid gland.

However, the patient can't lose weight, has difficulty concentrating, has dry skin, thin hair and eye brows, and is cold all the time—all classic signs of hypothyroidism. Why is this occurring? The receptor sites for the thyroid hormones have become resistant. This is called *type II hypothyroidism*.[2] The receptor site resistance is usually due to a nutritional deficiency and/or an environmental toxicity. It is important for the treating physician and the patient to understand that the sensitivity of receptors is every bit as important as the hormone levels for proper function to occur.

To summarize, the control of the production of the sex hormones and thyroid hormones is under the control of a negative feedback system under the control of the hypothalamus and pituitary. Both the level of hormone production and the receptor sensitivity of the cell membrane in the brain, muscles, bones, and skin are equally important for optimum body function. Lowered production of hormone and/or receptor resistance causes hypo-function. Therefore, an individual can experience symptoms of hypo-function of the thyroid, adrenals, or gonads even when hormone levels appear within reference range. Because the hormone levels fluctuate throughout a twenty-four hour cycle, the timing of the measurement of the hormones is important.

effect of ✱s tored pills ?

not understand

In the next chapter, you will learn how the hormones are made. A chart demonstrating the interrelationship of the hormones is below.

The Hormones Interrelationships
© Kelly Miller, DC NMD FASA FBAARM

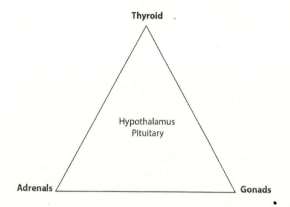

Chapter 2 References

1. Haring R, Volzke H, Stzveling A, et al. Low serum testosterone levels are associated with increased risk of mortality in a population-based cohort of men aged 20-70. *European Heart Journal. DOI: http://dx.doi.orgliv.110.1093/eurheartj/ehq009* First published online: 17 February 2010.
2. Starr M, *Hypothyroidism Type 2: The Epidemic Revised 2013 Edition*, Irvine, CA: New Voice Publications; 2005.

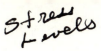

Most hormones are all made from the same source, cholesterol. There are three separate major groups of hormones manufactured from cholesterol. They are the *glucocorticoids* such as cortisol, the *mineralocorticoids* such as aldosterone, and the sex hormones such as testosterone and estrogen. The sex hormones include pregnenolone, progesterone, DHEA, testosterone, estrone (E1), estradiol (E2), and estriol (E3). Cortisol and aldosterone, also derived from cholesterol, are discussed later in this book.

People are often concerned about their cholesterol levels being too high. However, we should be just as concerned about our cholesterol levels being too low. Many labs use the reference range of 125-200 mg/dl for total cholesterol. However, there have been several studies demonstrating an increased morbidity rate in hospital patients with cholesterol levels below 165 mg/dl and an even greater morbidity rate for those with cholesterol levels below 145 mg/dl.[1,2] If your cholesterol levels are too low, it affects your ability to make hormones.

Two of the most common reasons for elevated cholesterol in the population are not from excess dietary cholesterol, but from an under-functioning thyroid, or excess sugar intake, especially of high fructose corn syrup. Inherited genetic patterns also play a role in almost 50 % of cases. However, it is lifestyle choices that cause the negative epigenetic expression, or heritable changes in gene expression. There are several gene patterns related to increased incidence of *VLDLs* (very low density lipoproteins, the small sticky kind) that are caused by increased sugar or alcohol intake or B vitamin deficiencies caused by lack of dietary intake. Like all things in the body, everything is about balance. I like to see cholesterol levels of 180-200 mg/dl for optimum hormone production, but consider levels 150-220 mg/dl normal.

The vast majority of cholesterol is manufactured in the liver. Cholesterol is first converted to pregnenolone, the "mother of all hormones."[2] This process occurs in the adrenal glands, specifically in the *mitochondria* (power plant) of the adrenal cortex cells. Pregnenolone has two potential pathways of conversion. It can either convert to progesterone, or it can convert to DHEA. Again, a specific enzyme accomplishes each conversion. In the other pathway, progesterone converts to either aldosterone or cortisol, each process controlled by an enzyme, but now occurring in what is known as the endoplasmic reticulum of the cells in either the cortex of the adrenals, or the gonads (testes or ovaries). The endoplasmic reticulum is a network of membranous tubules within the cytoplasm of a cell. See the illustration of a cell below. I realize this is a little detailed, but if you know this, you know more than most doctors.

Illustration of a cell

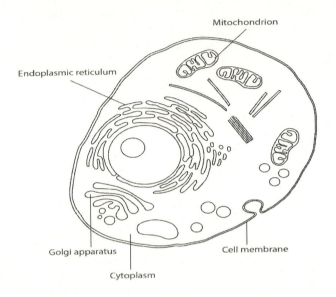

CELL

DHEA, known as the "father of all hormones," is the largest pool of hormones in the body and converts into two different intermediaries, androstenedione and androstenediol. Androstenedione converts to either testosterone or estrone (E1). The intermediary, androstenedione became well known a few years ago because of the professional baseball players who were using it. You may remember all those muscular guys breaking all the hitting records. Well, thanks to them, androstenedione is now a banned substance. Androstenedione and testosterone exist in a common pool together, where they transform back and forth as needed. Testosterone converts to estradiol (E2), and androstenedione can convert to cortisol, testosterone, or estrone (E1).

Estrone (E1) and estradiol (E2) exist in a common pool together, transforming back and forth as needed. The last step in the hormone process is to estriol (E3) from either estrone or estradiol. Once estriol (E3) is formed, it cannot convert back to either estrone (E1) or estradiol (E2). A picture is worth a thousand words. (See the Hormone Pathways illustration.)

The Hormone Pathways
© Kelly Miller, DC NMD FASA FBAARM

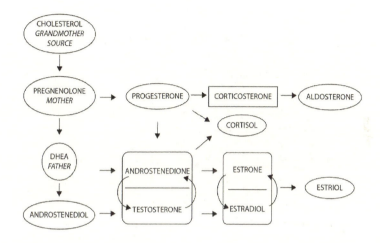

All of these conversions of one hormone to a new hormone require an enzyme that contains B vitamins and specific minerals. Nutritional deficiencies, genetic variances, and environmental and emotional stressors can create problems with the conversion of one hormone into another hormone. There are a number of genetic variances, particularly involving testosterone and estrogen that effect the conversion and the detoxification of these hormones. These conversions are covered in more detail in the individual chapter on each hormone.

Generally speaking, the more stress you have in your life the greater the negative impact on your various hormone levels. It is important to understand how this happens. As discussed earlier, pregnenolone converts to progesterone, which converts to cortisol. Cortisol production is our first line of defense against stress in our hormone system. The other pathway for pregnenolone is DHEA. DHEA is an anabolic (tissue building) hormone. Both progesterone and DHEA can convert to testosterone, which is also an anabolic (tissue building) hormone. When we are under a lot of stress (can't pay the bills, going through a divorce, get fired or laid off, lose a loved one, have an injury, don't get enough sleep, eat too much fast food, or consume too much coffee, soda, alcohol) our hormone system ramps up the production of cortisol. This cortisol production goes on non-stop until we reduce or eliminate the stress, or until our adrenals can no longer produce or keep up with adequate cortisol production. This acute or chronic cortisol production is at the expense of DHEA and testosterone. Instead of the pregnenolone converting to DHEA, it converts primarily to progesterone and then to cortisol. Therefore, all the anabolic hormones that build and repair our bodies are deficient. Over time, the progesterone and pregnenolone become depleted trying to make more cortisol. This is known as *pregnenolone steal.*[3] (See the illustration below.)

Pregnenolone Steal
The Adverse effects of Stress
© Kelly Miller, DC NMD FASA FBAARM

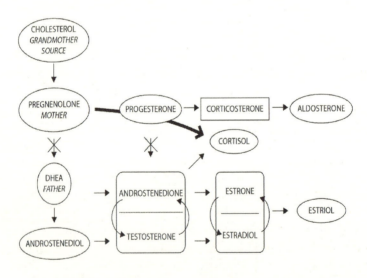

The fundamental concept that I want you to get is that there is no such thing as a single hormone deficiency. The cortisol connection is why some people get only temporary results with supplementation of testosterone or estradiol. The adrenal function, in this case the cortisol production, has to be corrected to achieve stabilization of the entire hormonal system. This is an often-overlooked component by many doctors offering bio-identical hormone therapy. See more information under the Cortisol chapter. To reiterate, cortisol is synonymous with stress. You can reduce stress levels by improving sleeping patterns, food intake, fluid intake, exercise, and thinking and by reducing environmental toxins, such as mercury and BPA.

Note: Stress levels

Everyone should know This

Chapter 3 References

1. Rauchhaus M, Clark A, Doehner W, et al. The relationship between cholesterol and survival on patients with chronic heart failure. *J Am Coll Cardiol* 2003;42(11):1933-1940. *doi.10.1016/j.jacc.2003.07.016.*

2. Horwich TB, Hernandez AF, Dai D, et al. Cholesterol levels and in-hospital mortality in patients with acute decompensated heart failure" *American Heart Journal,* 2008 Dec; 156, (6): 1170-1176

3. Pregnenolone Steal, 2016. https://www.functionalmedicineuniversity.com/members/login.cfm?hpage=forum%2Fopenthread.cfm%3Fforum%3D15%26threadid%3D2420&cfmbbthreadid=2420. Accessed 04/01/2015

Chapter 4: Liposome Technology and Why It Is so Important

"Liposome technology is the greatest breakthrough in the area of nutrition in the last decade, if not the last century." Dr. Paul Tai, President and Chairman of Brazil American Aging and Regenerative Medical Society.

All vitamin, mineral, herbal, and hormone supplements are not created equal. Generally speaking, you often get what you pay for. If you think your one-a-day vitamin is covering all your nutritional needs, you are sadly mistaken. There is absolutely no way you can supplement for all your deficiencies in one pill. If you could, the size of the pill would be golf-ball size. One-a-day vitamin/mineral pills are synthetic. The molecular structure of these synthetic vitamins is only a dysfunctional mirror image of natural vitamins. Natural vitamins exist in what is known as a *cis* formation, while synthetic vitamins exist in a *trans* formation.[1,2] These two designations refer to the relative orientation of certain elements in the molecule. Your body, specifically your cell membrane, knows the difference. The cell membranes are designed to use the cis formation, not the trans formation of the synthetic vitamin. This is like trying to wear your left shoe on your right foot. It just does not fit and doesn't work well.

Good natural multi-vitamin and anti-oxidant formulas usually require four to eight tablets per day, and they are fairly large in size. In my office, I recommend one formula for multi vitamin/minerals at two tablets B.I.D (two times each day) and another formulae for anti-oxidants of two tablets B.I.D.[3] I feel these formulas are as good as there is out there. However, they are not enough to meet the needs of everyone. How much of any given nutrient any individual needs is going to be dependent upon genes and lifestyle. Most of the common one-a-day vitamins sold are of no value, in my opinion.

The challenges with oral consumption of capsules or pills is getting through the digestive system, getting through the liver, and then getting through the cell membranes. You have heard the old adage that you are what you eat. The truth of the matter is you are what is absorbed through the cell membrane. This is not only true for vitamin, mineral, and antioxidant supplementation, but also for hormone supplementation. It is estimated, on average, that only five to ten percent of any given nutrient or hormone taken orally in pill form ever reaches the blood stream.[4] There are many variants in the ability of any given individual to digest, based on the individual's stomach, pancreas, liver, gallbladder, and small intestine function. In the case of hormones, if the dose is *supra physiological* (higher than the body's natural ability to make) the liver produces *SHBG* (sex hormone biding globulin) and indiscriminately binds all hormones, causing hormone levels to decline dramatically. Moreover, this process produces stress on an already overworked liver.

There are also gene variants that cause an individual to need much more of a specific nutrient or hormone than another or may require the nutrient to be in a certain form to pass through the cell membrane to be used. There are many common gene variants for specific vitamin, minerals, antioxidants, and hormones. For example, there is a gene variant called *MTHFR* related to a reduced ability to use folate/folic acid.[5] This may cause an individual to need fifty percent or more higher level of folate/folic acid in dietary intake than average. This genetic variant increases the likelihood of a deficiency to occur that can influence a multitude of increased risk factors for cleft palate, heart defect, learning and behavioral disabilities, breast cancer, gastrointestinal cancers, and dementia.[5] Therefore, absorption through the cell membrane of adequate amounts of nutrients is critical for optimal health.

The use of *sublingual* and *transdermal* supplementation has been around for several years. The advantages of sublingual supplementation is that is absorbed through the capillaries under the tongue and taken to cell membrane receptor sites, without going through the stomach and liver first. As a result, a much higher percentage of the nutrient reaches the cell membrane. Transdermal applications take advantage of capillary circulation to the cell membrane receptor sites, again bypassing the digestive system and liver. This allows for a much higher percentage of the nutrient or hormone to reach target cell receptor sites. The only limiting factor with transdermal applications is the carrier creams used to accompany the nutrient or hormone. Sublingual and transdermal technologies consistently produce better absorption of a product than conventional oral dosing.

Liposome technology greatly enhances the absorption of sublingual or transdermal products because of something called *phosphatidylcholine*.[6] Phosphatidylcholine is a naturally occurring lipid (fat) present in all cell membranes. In liposome technology, the nutrient or hormone is wrapped with the phosphatidylcholine. When the nutrient or hormone surrounded by the phosphatidylcholine, comes knocking on the door (cell membrane receptor site), the door is opened for the nutrient or hormone because it recognizes it as a friend (the nutrient or hormone binds with the receptor site and passes through the cell membrane). This is why liposome technology is extremely important and exciting. It facilitates the absorption of the nutrient or hormone into the cell by at least ten times the rate of the average oral supplementation. All of the transdermal hormones— pregnenolone, progesterone, DHEA, testosterone, estradiol and estriol—are now available with this technology. There are also many vitamins and antioxidants available with this technology as well, such as the B vitamins, D3/K2, superoxide dismutase, catalase, and glutathione.[3] Whenever possible, this technology is used for the supplements I recommend for my patients. This is important because it ensures that what you are taking is reaching the target cells and tissues.

1. Zechmeister L. *Cis-Trans Isomeric Carotenoids, Vitamin A and Arylpolyenes.* Atlanta, GA: Academic Press; 1962.

2. Ben-Anotz A, Levy Y. Bio-availability of a natural isomer compared with synthetic all-trans beta carotene in human serum. *Am J Clin Nutr* 1996 May; 63(5): 729-734.

3. Tai PL. *Encyclopedia of Natural Products*, Dearborn, Michigan: BARM PMA Publications, 2015.

4. Stabler SP, Allen RA. Vitamin B12 Is A World-Wide Problem , *Annual Review of Nutrition* , July 2004; 24: 295-326. *DOI:10.1146/annurev.nutr.24.012003.132440.*

5. Tai PL. *8 Powerful Secrets to Anti-Aging.* Dearborn, MI: Health Secrets; 2007.

Chapter 5: Cholesterol, the Source

is it understood ?
Vit D son

Many of you reading this book may be wondering why there is a chapter on cholesterol in a book about hormones. The answer is quite simple. All the glucocorticoids, mineralocorticoids, and sex hormones as well as Vitamin D are derived from cholesterol. Your testosterone and estrogen levels are dependent upon the cholesterol in the body.

There are probably few other topics where so much misinformation has been disseminated to doctors and the public. When I first started my practice in 1980, a normal cholesterol was considered to be 280 mg/dl or below. In 1986, the level was revised to a level of 240 mg/dl or below as normal. A few years later, the normal value for total cholesterol was set at 200 mg/dl or below. There is now a movement to push the normal value to 185 mg/dl and below. Achieving that level would increase prescription medications to at least thirty percent more of the American population. That sounds like a grand slam home run for the pharmaceutical companies that make statin medications. I can assure you that once the patents run out on all the statin drugs, there will be a revelation via commercials from the pharmaceutical companies that the new drugs developed for elevated cholesterol are better than the statins and that they have discovered that elevated cholesterol was not the total answer for the cause of coronary heart disease. It may come as no surprise to many that this theory of elevated cholesterol causing heart disease and attacks has been thoroughly disproven since the mid 1990's.

Additionally, there are disadvantages to taking statins. Erectile dysfunction and loss of libido are fairly common side effects from long-term statin use due to the interference of the body's conversion of cholesterol into pregnenolone. The majority of the cholesterol that is measured by blood serum tests is manufactured in the liver. Both cholesterol and triglycerides are by-products of sugar metabolism in the liver, especially the *VLDL* (very low density lipoprotein) cholesterol that sticks to your arteries. Large amounts of VLDLs are produced by high fructose corn syrup in sodas, high fructose levels in fruit juices, and by alcohol consumption. Approximately one-third of all the calories from fructose or alcohol are converted into VLDL cholesterol and stored fat. Yes, it is the sugar in your diet, not the fats, that is mainly responsible for your elevated cholesterol levels.

There is little difference in terms of the effect in the liver production of making VLDL's from equal caloric intake of soda vs. orange juice vs. alcohol. There is evidence that other negative side effects from statins are *congestive heart failure,*[1] *myopathy,*[2] *neuropathy,*[3,4,5] *cognitive loss,* [6] *dementia,*[6,7] *Alzheimer's,*[6] and possibly *A.L.S. (Amyotrophic Lateral Sclerosis, a.k.a. Lou Gehrig's disease).*[8] These complications appear to be due to the inhibition of an essential nutrient, *CoenzymQ10.* Statin medications interfere with the production of this essential nutrient. The fact of the matter is that more people are affected by the side effects of these drugs than benefit from taking them. One study on statin medication only demonstrated that 1.1 people out of one hundred (1.1 %) had decreased risk for heart attacks after taking the medication for three years.[9] On the other hand, there are several studies reporting patients who were admitted to hospitals with low cholesterol levels that later died, indicating there is an increased rate of morbidity with total cholesterol levels under 165 mg/dl and an even greater morbidity rate with the total cholesterol levels under 145 mg/dl.[10,11]

Why is this?

Once you understand that most of our hormones are manufactured from cholesterol, the morbidity associated with low cholesterol makes more sense. Low cholesterol means that a person is to have low pregnenolone, progesterone, DHEA, and testosterone levels because all these hormones originate from cholesterol. Therefore, optimum cholesterol levels are critical for optimum hormone production. Some elderly people may exhibit elevated cholesterol in their seventies, eighties, or nineties for the first time in their life. It is theorized by some that this is merely the body's attempt to make more hormones. This is possible, but it also could be secondary to problems with sugar metabolism in the elderly. For example, my mother never had an elevated cholesterol or blood sugar level until she was age ninety-two. This more likely than not occurred due to her sedentary lifestyle coupled with the starchy diet and desserts at the assisted living facility. Her doctor recommended a statin medication at age ninety-two while I have found no statistical data demonstrating the reduction of incidence of heart attacks or strokes for a person past the age of seventy who were placed on statins.[9] Yet, statins are routinely prescribed for patients in this age group by some doctors.

Most people have heard the negatives on elevated cholesterol. There are just as many <u>negatives on having cholesterol levels too low.</u> Like all things in the body, everything is about balance.

Note √í

Chapter 5 References

1. Ghierghiade M, Bonn RO. Chronic Heart Failure in the United States, A Manifestation of Coronary Artery Disease. *Circulation,* 1998 Jan; 97 (3): 282-9.
2. Mac Murray, JJ. Statins and chronic heart failure: do we need a large outcome study? *Am. Coll. Cardiol.* 2002; 39(10): 1567-1573. *DOI: 10.1016/So735-1097(02)01827-2.*
3. Voora D, Svati HS, Spasojevic I. The SL01B1 Genetic Variant is Associated with Statin-Induced Side Effects. *Am. Cardiol.* 2009; 54(17): 1609-1616. *DOI:.10.1016/j.jac2009.04.0543.*
4. Jeppien U, Crust D, Smith T, Sendriup SH. Statins and peripheral neuropathy. *European Journal of Clinical Pharmacol,* 1999; 54: 835-8.
5. Chong, PH, Boshivich, A, Sterkovic, N. Statin –Associated Peripheral Neuropathy: Review of the Literature. 2012 Jan 16. DOI: 10.1592/phco.24.13.1194.38084
6. Lieberman A, Lyons K, Levine J, Meyerburg R. Statins, Cholesterol, Co-Enzyme Q10, and Parkinson's Disease. *Parkinsonism Relat Disord,* 2005 Mar; 11 (2): 81-4.
7. Nilsson K, Gufstafson L. Hultberg B. Improvement of cognitive function after cobolamine/folate supplement in elderly patients with dementia and elevated plasma homocysteine. *Int J Geriatr Psychiatry,* 2001 Jun; 16 (6): 609-14.
8. Edwardy IR, Star K, Kiuri A. Statins, neuromuscular degenerative disease and amyotrophic lateral sclerosis-like syndrome. *Drug Safety,* 2007; 30 (6): 515-25.
9. Graveline D. *Statin Drugs Side-effects and the Misguided War on Cholesterol.* USA: Duane Graveline; 2004.
10. Horwich TB, Hernandez AF, Dai D, Yancy, CW, Fonarow GC. Cholesterol levels in a hospital mortality in patients with acute decompensated heart failure. *Am. Heart J.* 2008; 156(6); 1170-6.

√í *Very important*

11. Akerblom JL, Costa R, Luchsinger JA, et al. Relation of plasma lipids to all-cause mortality in Caucasian, African-American, and Hispanic elders. *Age and Ageing,* 2008 Mar; 37: 207-213.
12. Sinatra S, Bowden, J. *The Great Cholesterol Myth.* Beverly, MA: Fair Winds Press; 2012.
13. Tai, PL. *Clinical Nutrition.* Dearborn Heights, MI: Health Secrets USA; 2016
14. Cohen JS, *What You Must Know About Statin Drugs & Their Natural Alternatives.* Garden City Park, NY: Square One Publishers.

Chapter 6: Pregnenolone

Pregnenolone, which is converted from cholesterol in the mitochondria of the adrenal cortex, is known as the mother of all hormones. Dietary sources that can interfere with the conversion of cholesterol to pregnenolone are excess saturated fats and trans-fats.[1] Excess trans-fats are common in the *S.A.D.* (standard American diet). Since cholesterol is the source of all glucocorticoids—such as cortisol, mineralocorticoids like aldosterone, and the sex hormones, it is known as the "grandmother" of all hormones, Therefore, the indiscriminate use of statin drugs in an attempt to lower cholesterol can have a profound negative impact on the cascading of all hormone production. Pregnenolone is converted to one of two pathways, either to progesterone or DHEA. Progesterone then converts to cortisol or aldosterone and may also convert to testosterone. DHEA converts to testosterone or sometimes estrogen through intermediaries. DHEA represents the largest pool of hormone, and is known as the father of all the hormones. (See illustration below.)

The Hormone Pathways
Pregnenolone

© Kelly Miller, DC NMD FASA FBAARM

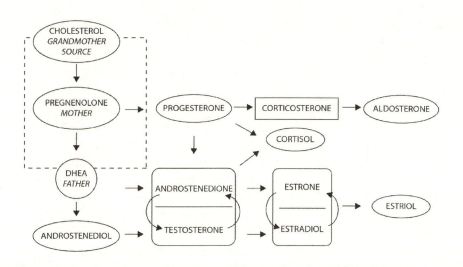

Pregnenolone improves excitation and inhibition of the nervous system, increases resistance to stress, improves physical and mental energy, increases nerve transmissions and memory, and reduces pain and inflammation.[1-6]

In 1943, Dr. Hans Selye, who is responsible for our modern awareness and terminology of stress, found that pregnenolone negated the damaging effects of excess cortisol, another hormone produced in the adrenal cortex that deals with stress and inflammation.[2] (See the chapter on cortisol.) Pregnenolone supplementation was able to neutralize the symptoms of excess cortisol that include depression, water retention, insomnia, overeating, weakened immunities, and destabilized liver functions.

Pregnenolone is also vital to the function of memory. Numerous studies through the years have shown with optimum levels of pregnenolone that one is able to think more clearly and with less delay in recalling information. Pregnenolone levels are optimum in most people at about age thirty-five.[6] Maintenance, with supplementation of pregnenolone that will achieve levels in the top quartile of reference range for a healthy thirty-five-year-old greatly reduces the risk for dementia, Alzheimer's, and senility. [6]

Pregnenolone supplementation has demonstrated very positive effects directly correlated with arthritis. It has been shown to reduce swelling, inflammation, and the joint and muscle pain associated with arthritis.[1,3] Pregnenolone supplementation has also been shown to be helpful with autoimmune diseases, such as lupus and psoriasis, and promise in the area of spinal cord injuries and multiple sclerosis.[1,3] It is helpful in the treatment of neuropathies involving the myelin sheath, the covering around the nerve.[1,3]

Symptoms of pregnenolone deficiency include loss of short-term memory, forgetfulness or fuzzy-thinking, depression, reduction of perceived brightness of color, and pessimism.[1] Again, now that we know that pregnenolone is dependent upon cholesterol, we can better understand why statin drugs that interfere with the synthesis of cholesterol and the conversion into pregnenolone leave so many users of this drug with CRS (Can't Remember Sh*t) Syndrome.

There are two areas for certain that pregnenolone supplementation can be helpful in aging—with thinking and helping to cope with stress. [1-6] The absolute best way to administer *exogenous* pregnenolone is through transdermal application utilizing liposome technology. *Liposome* technology is certainly the nutritional breakthrough of the decade, if not the century. Liposome technology involves the encapsulation of a nutrient or hormone with *phosphatidylcholine*. Phosphatidylcholine is a naturally occurring lipid (fat) that is contained within the cell membranes. Getting a nutrient or hormone through the cell membrane is the key to having that particular substance to be used by the cell. Just because a mineral, vitamin, or hormone is in the blood, does not mean it is getting inside the cell. The vitamin, mineral, or hormone must pass through the cell membrane to be used. Because the phosphatidylcholine is made up of the same substance found within the cell membrane, the cell accepts it more readily and allows passage of it through the cell membrane along with the nutrient or hormone accompanying it. Therefore, liposome is the best delivery system to date at helping to make a nutrient or hormone bio-available for the cell.

Below is a self-assessment to help you determine if you may have a pregnenolone imbalance. If you have symptoms in one of the columns, follow the advice at the top of the column.

PREGNENOLONE SELF-ASSESSMENT[1]
(Used with permission of author)

Pregnenolone Deficiency	Pregnenolone Excess
If supplementation has begun, increase dosage.	If supplementation has begun, decrease dosage.
loss of short term memory, forgetfulness	edginess, feeling uptight
fuzzy thinking	frequent worry
Depression	
Reduction in perceived brightness of colors	

Chapter 6 References

1. Yanick P. *Prohormone Nutrition*, Montclair, NJ: Longevity Institute International, 1998.
2. Tai, PL. *8 Powerful Secrets to Anti-Aging*. Dearborn Heights, MI: Health Secrets, USA; 2007.
3. Selye H, Clarke E. Potentiation of a pituitary extract with Δ^{5-} pregnenolone and additional observations concerning the influence of various organs or steroids, metabolism. *Review Canadienne Biologie,* 1943; 2 (3):319-28.
4. Regelson W. *The Super-Hormone Promise: Nature's Antidote to Aging.* New York: Pocket Books; 1996.
5. Flood, JF, Morely JE. Roberts E. Memory enhancing effect in male mice of pregnenolone and steroids metabolically derived from it. *Proceedings from the National Academy of Science the United States of America,* 1992; 89:1562.
6. Mc Garack TH. Chevalley J, Weisberg J. The use of pregnenolone in various clinical disorders. *Journal of Clinical Endocrinology and Metabolism,* 1951; 11:559-77.
7. Roberts E. Pregnenolone from Seyle to Alzheimer's. *Biochem. Pharma,* 1995; 48 (1): 1-16.

Chapter 7: Progesterone

Progesterone is converted from pregnenolone in the *endoplasmic reticulum* of the ovary. Progesterone cascades down to make the *glucocorticoids* like cortisol and the mineralocorticoids, corticosterone, and aldosterone. It also can convert to testosterone. See the hormone pathways chart.

The Hormone Pathways
Progesterone

© Kelly Miller, DC NMD FASA FBAARM

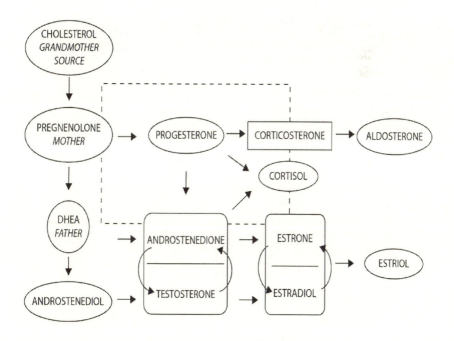

Progesterone is the synergistic balancing counterpart to estrogen, specifically estradiol (E2). Progesterone gives protection to the breast, uterus, and ovaries from cancer, helps bone growth, reduces heart disease, and gives peace of mind. It is the hormone that supports conception and sustains pregnancy. Progesterone has been called *the woman's friend.* In a normal menstrual cycle, progesterone levels rapidly increase with ovulation, occurring approximately fourteen days after menstruation begins. Progesterone levels usually peak at day 21 and rapidly drop off day 28. Progesterone, like estrogen, has both a negative and positive feedback system to the hypothalamus and pituitary. The positive feedback system is to maintain sustained levels of progesterone after ovulation takes place until the shedding of the uterine lining should pregnancy not occur. See HPG Axis illustration.

Hypothalamus-Pituitary-Gonads (HPG) Axis

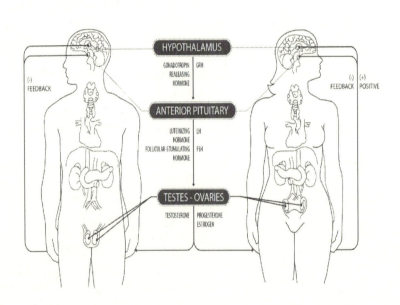

Progesterone promotes pro-gestation and functions as a natural diuretic that blocks *aldosterone* (a hormone that helps us retain sodium [salt]). It uses fat for energy and is a natural anti-depressant and anti-anxiety. It also may increase libido, and it promotes cell differentiation, splits and duplicates into two daughter cells, and prevents blood clots. Again, progesterone is a major protector of the breast, uterus, and ovaries and from uterine fibroids and endometriosis.[1-8]

Generally speaking, if a woman is having a lot of negative symptoms in the first fourteen days of her cycle, it is usually related to estrogen levels. Negative symptoms in the last fourteen days are usually related to progesterone. Ninety percent of women in America have problems in the last fourteen days. Additionally, the incidence of breast cancer is forty percent greater in women with a progesterone deficiency. Transdermal progesterone has been shown to decrease breast cell growth by four hundred percent. It is interesting to note that there is twenty times more progesterone in the brain than in the blood serum, which explains its profound mood calming, relaxing effect.[1]

Some of the primary symptoms of progesterone deficiency are the following: anxiety, depression, irritability, mood swings, insomnia, pain and inflammation, *osteoporosis*, amenorrhea, PMS, cystic breasts, painful breasts, water retention, craving for chocolate and sweets, postpartum depression, miscarriage, infertility, swelling of the belly, hands, and feet, headaches before menstruation, excessive menstruation, uterine fibroids, and endometriosis.[1,6,8] Progesterone deficiency is common in women. Some of the common causes of progesterone deficiency are the following: stress (which causes increased cortisol production), anti-depressant medications, excessive *arginine* (an amino acid synthesized by the body) consumption, sugar, excessive saturated fat, deficiencies in vitamins A, B$_6$, C, zinc, and decreased thyroid function.[1,2,8]

Women experience their first mild decline in progesterone levels at about age thirty to thirty-five. This drop in progesterone levels is the primary reason women have difficulty sustaining pregnancies when they approach age forty and beyond. Women usually experience their first mild drop in estrogen levels at age forty to forty-five. Progesterone levels drop again markedly at the onset of menopause and continue to decline. Estrogen levels also drop at menopause, but not as much as progesterone levels. As stated previously, approximately ninety percent of women suffer with symptoms of PMS, but fortunately ninety percent have a positive response from transdermal progesterone therapy. Men produce progesterone in the adrenals while women produce progesterone in their ovaries. Progesterone's main effect in men is its conversion into testosterone and balancing the negative effects of estrogen.

The modern day guru on progesterone is Dr. John R. Lee, authoring tens of peer-reviewed publications as well as several books on progesterone. Dr. Lee was also a proponent for the use of bio-identical transdermal progesterone for his patients. Natural bio-identical progesterone is not the same as the synthetic prescription *Progestin*, however, so don't be confused by these two. Natural bio-identical supplementation is exactly in the same form as the body makes it. Natural bio-identical progesterone has one hundred percent receptor activity while the synthetic prescription, Progestin, has an eight percent receptor activity. This is because the molecular structure of progesterone was altered in order to patent it as a drug. Because it is altered, the receptors do not respond the same to the Progestin as they do with natural progesterone. An analogy to this would be that you possessed a skeleton key that would only unlock eight of the one hundred potential doors in a house instead of having the actual key made for all one hundred doors. Progestin is an extraterrestrial molecule that is not naturally designed for your receptor sites. It plays havoc with the body by creating problems locally at the receptor sites and challenges in dealing with its elimination from the body.

Progesterone Deficiency/Fibroids Case History

T.E. was a forty-five-year-old female who I had originally treated for a severely herniated lumbar disc. She was having lower back pain with radiation, numbness, and weakness in her leg. This fully resolved without surgery in about eight to twelve weeks, and she was able to return to normal activities. I had also treated her father nutritionally for congestive heart failure and a wound from abdominal surgery that had not resolved for months. His abdominal wound healed in about thirty to forty-five days after supplementation of appropriate nutraceuticals. T.E. told me that she had multiple breast lumps and fibroids, and she was concerned about the possibility of surgeries for these. She indicated that she had heavy bleeding with cramps for two to three days with anxiousness during her menstrual cycle. She also had complaints of a loss of libido. I recommended a saliva hormone test as I suspected a severe progesterone deficiency.

The saliva hormone test revealed a severe progesterone deficiency as well as low cortisol (indicating adrenal fatigue), DHEA, and testosterone. You may recall I have said there is no such thing as a single hormone deficiency. You may also recall that cortisol inhibits DHEA and subsequent testosterone production. TSH levels were over 2 mIU/L, which suggested possible low thyroid function. Basal body temperature readings averaged 96.8 (normal 98.6) confirming a type II hypothyroid condition. It is always important to know how the thyroid is working because it has a direct influence on the ovaries in the production of estrogen and progesterone. You will learn more about this when you read the thyroid chapter. T.E. was given recommendations for supplements to support both the adrenals and the thyroid daily. In addition, she was given transdermal pregnenolone and DHEA daily and progesterone only on days fifteen through twenty-eight of her menstrual cycle. By the time her next menstrual cycle started, T.E. reported less cramping, breast tenderness, and anxiousness. She reported her libido returned within two weeks after starting her supplementation. In fact, she was so impressed with her progress that she referred her husband. She continued her program and was re-tested at three months. It is important to re-test in two to three months after the initial tests to make sure dosing is optimal. Adjustments were made on dosing as indicated by her symptoms, how she was feeling as well as the test results. Her breast lumps continued to shrink except for the largest cyst. After six months, she elected to have this one cyst removed and has not had any reoccurrence of cysts in over two years. This has given her great peace of mind. During this time, she has achieved and maintained a ten- to twelve-pound weight loss and a ten percent body fat loss and has a new wardrobe two sizes smaller. This patient was always aware of her enlarged uterus from the fibroids, being able to feel it when she lay down on her back and palpated her lower abdomen. After about a year of treatment, she called me up and told me she could no longer feel it.

Case Study of Osteoporosis, Vaginal Dryness, Low Cortisol, Progesterone, and DHEA

B.A. was a pretty, petite sixty-eight-year-old woman who was concerned about her osteoporosis. She also reported a history of surgically resolved colon cancer over five years prior and a history of osteoporosis for ten years. Additionally, she walked on the treadmill and lifted weights three days each week. Her other complaint was that sexual intercourse was painful due to a lack of lubrication. She had been on Fosamax (medication prescribed to help osteoporosis) for a year but had discontinued it (rightfully so) after reading information about the potential side effects. Fosamax has been linked to causing *esophagitis* and bone destruction in the body. It has a *half-life* of ten years. If you have an adverse reaction, there is not much that can be done for it because it stays in your system for a very long time. Most of the drugs prescribed for *osteopenia* or osteoporosis work by inhibiting the activity of osteoclasts (cells that take out old bone cells). The drugs do not do anything to promote osteoblastic activity (new bone growth). However, that is exactly what natural progesterone does.

There was one other medication that she had been placed on for several years, Levothyroxine for her thyroid. She reports she did not feel any more energetic after being prescribed the medication, which is common among patients I have interviewed. *Hypothyroidism* is more common in women than men and increases in incidence after age sixty. She reported she had been placed on bio-identical progesterone in the past but had started some spotting. Because of this, she had discontinued its use. Apparently the prescribing doctor did not tell her that she would more likely than not have a few days of bleeding. This occurs commonly in menopausal women because the majority of women have been progesterone deficient for years before menopause and built up excess thickening of the uterine tissue because of the higher estrogen levels. This bleeding occurs until the excess tissue sheds. The progesterone deficiency is the reason that about forty percent of women have fibroids by *peri-menopause*. You may recall from the progesterone chapter that progesterone levels decline at age thirty to thirty-five in most women.

She was given a saliva hormone kit to take home, and she was asked to record her basal body temperature readings for five mornings. A genetic test for osteoporosis-related gene variants was deferred. Three gene variants—one for estrogen, one for Vitamin D, and one for *Interleukin-6* (an inflammatory marker) were assessed in this panel to determine if any of these could be a contributing factor to the development of osteoporosis. Her initial test results are below.

Miller Clinic for Optimal Health - SALIVARY BIOLOGICAL TEST REPORT

Report Date: 9/5/2014
Date Received: 9/3/2014

Patient Information
Last Menstrual Cycle: post-menopausal
Submitter Information
Institute: Miller Clinic for Optimal Health
Name: BA
Age of Menopause: 58
Address: 11804A North 56th Street
Date of Birth: 5/5/1946
Hx of Surgery:
Temple Terrace, FL 33617
Sex: F
Physician: Dr. Kelly Miller
Sample Collection Date: 8/28/2014
Medications:
Phone:
Sample ID No.: 14-00723
Send Lab Results To: Dr. Kelly Miller

HORMONE	LAB RESULT	FEMALE RANGE				MALE RANGE			Recommendation
		REFERENCE RANGE	ASSESSED OPTIMUM RANGE WITH SUPPLEMENT	ASSESSED OPTIMUM RANGE WITH TRANSDERMAL		REFERENCE RANGE	ASSESSED OPTIMUM RANGE WITH SUPPLEMENT	ASSESSED OPTIMUM RANGE WITH TRANSDERMAL	
Progesterone pg/ml Reportable Range 10-8000 pg/mL	292	Follicular 1/14 days 28-82; Luteal 15/28 days 127-446; Post Menopause 18-51	100-2500	200-5000		<26	20-100	200-2500	
Estrone pg/mL Reportable Range 1.4 - 300 pg/mL	>300	3-20	N/A	N/A		3-6	N/A	N/A	
Estradiol pg/ml Reportable Range 1.3-300 pg/mL	189.2	Follicular 5-9; Peak Max 12-20; Luteal 3-7; Post Menopause 1.5-3	10-20	20-100		<2.5	N/A	N/A	
Estriol pg/ml Reportable Range 1.0-1200 pg/mL	14.0	2-25	10-50	20-250		NA	NA	NA	
RATIO Progesterone/Estradiol	<2	Optimum Ratio of Progesterone / Estradiol ≥ 20 (For Female only)							
RATIO Estriol/Estradiol	0.0	Optimum Ratio of Estriol / Estradiol ≥ 4 (For Female only)							
Testosterone pg/ml Reportable Range 8.2 - 2000 pg/mL	133.7	AGE 20-29 45-49; 30-39 40-45; 40-49 35-40; 50-59 30-35; 60-69 25-30	40-60; 40-60; 40-60; 40-60; 40-60	100-300; 100-300; 100-300; 100-300; 100-300		145-155; 140-145; 135-140; 130-135; 125-130	140-165; 140-165; 140-165; 140-165; 140-165	250-2000; 250-2000; 250-2000; 250-2000; 250-2000	
DHEA pg/ml Reportable Range 1.0-2000 pg/mL	258.5	AGE 20-29 270-300; 30-39 240-270; 40-49 210-240; 50-59 180-210; 60-69 150-180; 70-79 120-150; Over 80 80-120	250-300; 250-300; 250-300; 250-300; 250-300; 250-300; 250-300	300-3000; 300-3000; 300-3000; 300-3000; 300-3000; 300-3000; 300-3000		300-330; 270-300; 240-270; 210-240; 180-210; 150-180; 100-150	300-350; 300-350; 300-350; 300-350; 300-350; 300-350; 300-350	350-3500; 350-3500; 350-3500; 350-3500; 350-3500; 350-3500; 350-3500	
CORTISOL nmol/L Reportable Range 0.09-19.8 nmol/L		ASSESSED OPTIMUM RANGE						ASSESSED OPTIMUM RANGE	
1st hour	8.67	13-18						13-18	
4th hour		6-9						6-9	
7th hour		3-6						3-6	
10th hour		2-3						2-3	
13th hour	2.62	1-2						1-2	

STOP SUPPLEMENT 24 HRS. PRIOR TO SALIVA SAMPLE

Comments: Miller Clinic for Optimal Health BIOLOGICAL report. This report reflects the optimal level of hormones that you may want to attain and maintain in order to have the healthy hormone levels of a 20-30 year old person.

The assessed range & optimum ranges are theoretical & to be used as a guide only by a health professional. Clinical symptoms must be monitored for drug or supplement dose adjustment to each individual needs. See your health professional for diagnosis, consultation & treatment.

DISCLAIMER
Results are not intended to diagnose and should be interpreted with the help of a physician or health care professional.

BA saliva report.xls

page 1 of 2

As suspected, her cortisol levels were low as adrenal dysfunction always accompanies hypothyroidism. In addition, her progesterone, estriol, and estrone levels were very low. Her estradiol levels were very high, and her estrone levels were above the reference range for testing. I was very concerned that her progesterone and estriol levels were not giving her adequate protection to offset the high estrone/estradiol levels, which increased her risk for breast, ovarian, and uterine cancers. Her progesterone and estriol levels needed to increase dramatically to compensate for her high estradiol/estrone levels. She was given recommendations for transdermal progesterone and high potency liquid extract of *Peuraria Mirifica*, an herb from Thailand.

In purchasing herbs, you must know what you are doing. You need to know what part of the plant has the medicinal component you are seeking, how it is prepared, and the concentration level of the extract. With herbs, you get what you pay for. If you find herbs that are priced much lower than most, they are probably the wrong part of the plant or the concentration level is low. I use pharmaceutical grade herbal extracts at the potency that was used in the scientific studies that demonstrated their efficacy. Many times a patient will try to find a product on-line that is less expensive only to find out it doesn't work, or they have to take three to five times more tablets or liquid to get the same effect. In the end, they are actually paying more. Until you become an expert in this area, follow the advice of an expert.

I also recommended that B.A. take a sublingual liquid B vitamin supplement and an estrogen detoxification formula that encouraged more 2-hydroxyestrone metabolite production as well as an herbal-based nutraceutical that gives localized cellular protection to the tissues containing the most estrogen receptors to offset her extremely high levels of estrone and estradiol. In addition, I recommended an adrenal support, co-factors for the conversion of T4 to T3, and 10,000 IU of liquid sublingual *D3/K2* for anti-oxidant protection and bone density. I instructed her to expect some cyclic bleeding for a little while because of the low progesterone and high estrogen levels. Estrogen is a tissue proliferator (makes tissue grow). Therefore, the uterus had become thickened. Once progesterone was made available, her body would get rid of the excess.

In the follow-up in two weeks, she reported mild spotting. This bleeding continued intermittently for about eight weeks and stopped as it always does once the excess tissue in the uterus is gone. She reported less pain with intercourse. Two weeks later, this complaint was resolved. Her energy was good and she was sleeping well. She continued the same therapy for two more weeks. At the end of that time, her progesterone and estriol levels were much higher, providing balance and protection against the excess estrone/estradiol. DHEA and testosterone and Vitamin D levels were elevated, all of which also encouraged increased bone density along with the progesterone.

Take the progesterone self-assessment test to help determine if your progesterone levels are optimal. If you have symptoms in one column, follow the advice at the top of that column.

PROGESTERONE SELF-ASSESSMENT [1]
(Used with permission of author)

Progesterone Deficiency	**Progesterone Excess**
If supplementation has begun, increase dosage.	If supplementation has begun, decrease dosage.
Premenstrual symptoms	Hot flashes worse W man.
Depression, mood swings, anxiety, nervousness, irritability	Increased cortisol
Breast swelling	Decreased glucose tolerance
Bloating, water retention	Increased fat storage
Uterine fibroids	Increased appetite/carbohydrate craving
Endometriosis	Depression
Excessive menstrual bleeding	"Drunk" feelings
Decreased HDL	Drowsiness
Insomnia	

1. Tai, PL. *8 Powerful Secrets of Anti-Aging*. Dearborn Heights, MI: Health Secrets USA; 2007.
2. Lauersen N. *PMS: Premenstrual Syndrome and You*. Wellington, NZ: Pinnacle Books; 1984.
3. Lee JR. Osteoporosis reversal of transdermal progesterone. *Lancet* 1990; 336:1327.
4. Tai, PL. *8 Powerful Secrets of Anti-Aging*. Dearborn Heights, MI: Health Secrets USA; 2005.
5. Lauersen N. *PMS: Premenstrual Syndrome and You*. Wellington, NZ: Pinnacle Books; 1984.
6. Lee JR. Osteoporosis reversal of transdermal progesterone. *Lancet,* 1990; 336: 1327.
7. Barret-Connor E, Stone S, Greendale G et al. PEDI (Postmenopausal Estrogen Progestin Intervention) Trials. *Maturitas.* 1997 Jul: 27 (3): 261-74.
8. Smidt IU, Wakley GK, Turner RT. Effects of estrogen on tibia histomorphometry in growing rats. *Calcif Tissue Int,* 2000; 67: 47-52.
9. Brownstein D, *Overcoming Thyroid Disorder.* West Bloomfield, MI: Med. Alton. Press; 2002.
10. Shairer C. The risk of breast cancer increase nearly 80% after 10 years of estrogen-progesterone (synthetic progesterone) and 160% after 20 years. *JAMA,* 2000, 283:688-691.
11. Laux M. *Natural Woman, Natural Menopause*, NY: HarperCollins; 1997.
12. Lee JR, Hopkins V. *What Your Doctor May Not Tell You About Breast Cancer.* New York: Warner Books; 2003.
13. Lee JR, Zava D, Hopkins V. *What Your Doctor May Not Tell You About Menopause.* New York: Warner Books; 2004.
14. Lee JR, Handly J, Hopkins V. *What Your Doctor May Not Tell You About Premenopause.* New York: Warner Books; 1999.
15. Lee JR, Hopkins V. *Hormone Balance Made Simple.* New York: Warner Books; 2006.
16. Lee JR. *Hormone Balance for Men.* New York: Warner Books; 2006.

Chapter 8: Cortisol

Without cortisol, our cells could not work. They could not transport materials through the cell membrane, make energy in the mitochondria, and replicate. Cortisol is converted from progesterone. (See Hormone Pathways in previous chapter.) Cortisol is produced in the adrenal cortex and is a glucocorticoid. There are three major classes of hormones produced in each of the three different zones of the adrenal cortex. The three classes of hormones are the mineralocorticoids, glucocorticoids, and the sex hormones. The outermost layer of the adrenal cortex is called the *zona glomerulosa* and produces aldosterone. The middle layer is called the *zona fasciculate* and produces cortisol. The innermost layer is the *zona reticularis* where DHEA and androstenedione are manufactured.

Illustration of Adrenal Gland

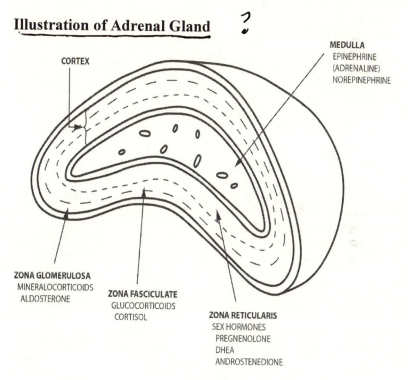

CORTEX

MEDULLA
EPINEPHRINE
(ADRENALINE)
NOREPINEPHRINE

ZONA GLOMERULOSA
MINERALOCORTICOIDS
ALDOSTERONE

ZONA FASCICULATE
GLUCOCORTICOIDS
CORTISOL

ZONA RETICULARIS
SEX HORMONES
PREGNENOLONE
DHEA
ANDROSTENEDIONE

Adrenal Gland

Cortisol is produced and secreted because of ACTH (adrenocorticotropic hormone), which is secreted by the pituitary gland. The pituitary gland secretes ACTH because the hypothalamus secretes a corticotrophin-releasing hormone that commands the pituitary to do so. The hypothalamus initiated this action because it is responsible for monitoring all internal sensory data in the body and recognizes that there is a need for more cortisol. This is called the H-P-A (hypothalamus-pituitary-adrenal) axis. It is the same negative feedback system that was discussed in Chapter 2. An increased need for cortisol is triggered after we eat, after we exercise, or during an emergency, either real or perceived. Once adequate amounts of cortisol are produced to handle the situation, cortisol receptors in the hypothalamus down-regulate the releasing hormone, which in turn reduces the ACTH production and secretion from the pituitary.

Cortisol is called a glucocorticoid because it mobilizes glucose (sugar) to the blood so we can have the energy we need to handle life. Responding to an emergency is referred to as a flight/fight response. This is when we are getting ready to fight the saber tooth tiger or run for the hills. Cortisol is also an anti-inflammatory that can create or remove bone mass from the body. If you have chronic cortisol production, you have too much glucose (because you are not really fighting or running from the tiger), and it is deposited as fat around your stomach as love handles and around internal organs.

Cortisol levels are highest between 6-8 AM, about forty-five minutes after rising, and are at the lowest at midnight. Levels generally trend down throughout the day, but rise a little after each meal and after exercise. However, people who work the night shift have their cortisol levels the highest whenever they wake up in the late morning or early afternoon, and then the levels quickly drop off.

Cortisol levels correlate positively with stress levels. Stress has been proven to contribute to heart disease, high blood pressure, colitis, irritability, rheumatism, depression, migraine headaches, diabetes, hardening of the arteries, and insomnia. Stress contributes to fatigue, sex problems, skin problems, allergies, overeating, asthma, kidney disease, ulcers, breathing difficulties, and increased smoking. Stress results in consistently high cortisol levels, which leads to poor health, obesity, excessive retention of water, loss of muscle tone, and loss of immune function with frequent illness. One of the reasons this occurs is that when cortisol production is ramped up it causes interference with DHEA and testosterone production. When we are under lots of stress, the vast majority of the pregnenolone is converted to progesterone and then to cortisol instead of going through the DHEA-testosterone pathway. This is known as pregnenolone steal. (See the Pregnenolone Steal Chart in Chapter 3.)

The body's ability to produce cortisol and its response with cortisol to stress, changes with age.[1-4] When we are younger, we have milder spikes of cortisol related to stress. As we age, our cortisol response is greater and lasts longer. A rapid lowering of cortisol after a stress ends is a big part of being healthy. Prolonged cortisol excess associated with chronic stress has been shown to have negative effects, such as impaired cognitive performance, reduced thyroid function, blood sugar imbalances, decreased bone density, sleep disruption, decreased muscle mass, elevated blood pressure, lowered immune function, slow wound healing, and increased body fat. If you have a prolonged high production of cortisol, you will eventually have disease while experiencing emotional disturbances. You will undoubtedly exhibit the side effects of too much cortisol, such as a moon-face, a buffalo hump, obesity, wrinkled skin, and weak muscles. These are all symptoms of *Cushing's disease*, the most prevalent disorder involving the glucocorticoids.

Once adrenal fatigue occurs from excess cortisol levels, this leads to a significantly lower secretion rate of cortisol by twenty-five to thirty percent in the elderly person.[1] It has been my personal experience that the vast majority of my patients over the age of forty have some degree of adrenal fatigue, causing lower cortisol levels. It's my opinion that the vast majority of middle-aged Americans are likewise suffering from some degree of adrenal fatigue. Factors that reduce cortisol include magnesium, Vitamin C, omega 3's, music therapy, massage, sexual intercourse, and laughing. Conversely, factors that increase cortisol levels are caffeine, sleep deprivation, severe stress, trauma, or prolonged physical exercise.

Cortisol imbalance is an often-overlooked factor by many doctors who offer bio-identical therapy. It is an absolutely essential component of the endocrine (hormone) system that must be addressed in order to achieve balance to the sex hormones.

Take this Stress Test to determine if you are at risk for excess stress and cortisol. Never or not is 0 point. Occasionally is 1 point. Frequently or yes is 2 points.[2] *interesting*

Stress Test

1. How often do you experience stressful situations?
2. How often do you feel tired or fatigued for no apparent reason?
3. How often do you get less than 8 hours of sleep? ✓
4. How often do you feel anxious or depressed?
5. How often do you feel angry or aggressive?
6. How often do you feel anxious or inadequate?
7. How often do you feel overwhelmed or confused?
8. How often is your sex drive lower than you would like it?
9. Do you tend to gain weight easily?
10. Are you currently dieting?
11. How often do you attempt to control your body weight?
12. How often do you get sick, catch cold, flu?
13. How often do you pay close attention to the foods you eat?
14. How often do you crave carbohydrates (sweets and breads)?
15. How often do you experience difficulty with memory or concentration?
16. How often do you experience digestive problem such as gas, bloating, ulcers, heartburn, constipation, or diarrhea?
17. How often do you experience tension headache or muscle tightness in your neck, shoulder or jaw?
18. Do you have high cholesterol (greater than 200mg/dl)?
19. Do you have high glucose (greater than 100 mg/dl) fasting?
21. Do you have high blood pressure (greater than 140/90 mm/hg)?

Score	Stress Level	Comment
0-5	Relaxed Jack/Low Risk	You are as cool as a cucumber. You either have a very low level of stress or a tremendous ability to deal effortlessly with incoming stresses.

6-10	Strained Jane/Moderate Risk	You may be suffering from overactive stress response and elevated cortisol levels and should incorporate anti-stress strategies into your lifestyle whenever possible, but don't stress about it.
>10	High Risk	You are almost definitely suffering from an overactive stress response and chronically elevated levels of cortisol. You need to take immediate steps to regain control.

One revelation I had recently is that much, if not most, of the stress in our lives is often self-imposed because of a loss of perspective about what is really important. We spend too much of our time and thoughts on things that do not really matter and worry needlessly about them. We have lost or forgotten our priorities. These wrong priorities cause fear and worry that cause chronic cortisol production, which eventually leads to disease. Re-establishing a sound Spirit-Mind-Body priority system goes a long way in way in reducing stress and helping to ensure a qualitative longevity. I have found these Biblical passages helpful for that.

For God has not given us a spirit of fear, but of power and of love and of a sound mind. II *Timothy 1:7.*

Which of you by worrying can add one cubit to his stature? *Matthew 6:27.*

Therefore do not worry about tomorrow, for tomorrow will worry about its own things. Sufficient for the day is its own trouble. *Matthew 6:34.*

We are often afraid or worry unnecessarily that we are going to lose our job, our status, or some of our material things. Here is what the Bible has to say about those worries.

There is no fear in love; but love casts out fear, because fear involves torment. But he who fears has not been made perfect in love.

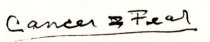

I John 4:18.

The good news is that we have the capability of monitoring our own thoughts.

Now faith is the substance of things hoped for, the evidence of things not seen. Hebrews 11:1.

Casting down arguments and every high thing that exalts itself against the knowledge of God, bringing every thought into captivity to the obedience of Christ. 2 Corinthians 10:5.

More importantly, we have the ability to change our priorities and our thinking.

And do not be transformed to this world, but be transformed by the renewing of your mind, that you may prove what is that good and acceptable and the perfect will of God. Romans 12:2.

Finally, brethren, whatever things are true, whatever things are noble, whatever things are just, whatever things are pure, whatever things are lovely, whatever things are of good report, if there is any virtue and if there is anything praiseworthy-meditate on these things. Philippians 4:8.

There are over 1,200 studies in peer-reviewed journals demonstrating the increased longevity of individuals who have a strong sense of faith.[5]

The Case of Self-Imposed Adrenal Fatigue

T.M. was a forty-one-year-old male who owned a physical therapy and fitness center, and he *looked fit*. He had good muscle mass and definition and had under ten percent body fat. His primary and immediate goals were to increase energy and muscle mass. His long-term goals were to have quality longevity and reduce his risks for cancer as both sides of his family had a history of cancer incidence. His diet was fairly good with eating fruits and vegetables daily, and his protein content was about thirty percent of total caloric intake. If anything, he may have been a little light on percentage of good quality fats. He lifted weights four to five days per week. He indicated he was a little stressed about work as many small business owners are. The most significant problem I saw with his lifestyle was that he was not getting enough sleep. He reported that he arose at 4:15 AM every morning, went to sleep 10:00 PM to 10:30 PM, and woke up once or twice every night but usually went back to sleep quickly. This meant he was averaging less than six hours of sleep each night. This amount of sleep is a problem for ninety-nine percent of the population. There are many epidemiological studies that indicate less than six hours of sleep each night reduce longevity by five to ten years. It has been my experience that this lack of sleep adversely affects the adrenal glands. Most people need seven and a half to eight and a half hours of sleep each night for optimum wellness.

After his consultation I took a sample of DNA from his inner cheeks for genetic testing for variants that could increase risks for certain cancers and gave him a saliva hormone test kit to take home. He was scheduled to return in two weeks to go over the test results with him. I emphasized the need for more sleep.

The saliva hormone test results confirmed my suspicion of adrenal dysfunction. His cortisol levels were 26.42 nmol/L (reference range 13-18 nmol/L, ideal 16-18 nmol/L) the first thing in the morning and 2.38 nmol/L (reference range 1-2 nmol/L) in the evening. His DHEA levels tested results were 91.7 pg/ml (reference range 210-240 pg/ml for 40-49 year olds). His DHEA levels were consistent with an average person who is eighty plus—not a good thing. The increased cortisol and decreased DHEA levels indicated he was in the second stage of adrenal fatigue. The next stage was adrenal exhaustion, meaning that his adrenal cortex that produces cortisol and DHEA was going into exhaustion if he did not get more sleep. Other significant readings were that his estrone levels were elevated at 35.7 pg/ml (reference range 3-6 pg/ml). This indicated he was converting too much of the intermediate androstenedione into estrone instead of testosterone. (See Sex Hormone Pathways in Chapter One.) His basal body temperature readings were acceptable, averaging 98.1 F (normal 98.6), indicating his thyroid metabolism was normal. Increased cortisol production inhibits the conversion of pregnenolone into DHEA as the vast majority of his pregnenolone was being converted into cortisol. This is known as pregnenelone steal and is covered in Chapter Six.

I recommended that he get an additional ninety minutes of sleep each night. I also recommended an adrenal support nutraceutical as well as transdermal pregnenolone and DHEA, a natural aromatase inhibitor to encourage more testosterone production and less production of estrone and 2-hydoxyestrone, and a liquid sublingual B vitamin supplement for methylation of 16-alpha-hydroxyestrone and 4-hydroxyestrone metabolites. In addition, liquid sublingual liposome supplements of Vitamins D3/K2, and anti-oxidants superoxide dismutase, catalase, and glutathione to help with genetic variants found in the DNA testing. He was advised to follow this schedule for the next three months when he would be re-tested. He was seen monthly in the interim and indicated he was being compliant except for missing DHEA application occasionally.

The saliva hormone test revealed that the estrone levels were markedly reduced at 13.6 pg/ml (reference range 3-6 pg/ml), down from 35.7 pg/ml, which means that his body was now producing less estrogen and estrogen metabolites due to the natural aromatase inhibitor he was taking. Unfortunately, his cortisol levels had only dropped down to 6.77 nmol/L (reference range 13-18 nmol/L) first thing in the morning and his DHEA levels were even lower than his previous test. When questioned about his sleep patterns, he admitted that he had made no changes and had been hit and miss with his DHEA applications.

What you need to understand is that a non-compliance issue for someone who has these readings can literally cost them their life. When cortisol and DHEA levels are low, the protective mucous lining called *secretory IgA* becomes thinner and the *tight junctions* of the single layer epithelial cells of the small intestine become loose. This combination of events increases the likelihood of the person developing a *leaky gut,* causing food/chemical allergy/sensitivity because of undigested food particles and microbes passing through the lining of the small intestine with subsequent inflammatory or immune reactions. The purpose of this secretory IgA is that it provides a mucous barrier, engulfing foreign invaders and depositing them outside your body with the stool. The loss of SIgA and loosening of the tight junctions can also lead to development of autoimmune disease.

Low cortisol and DHEA levels are hazardous to your health. The adrenal cortex produces both cortisol and DHEA. The lowering of these hormones signifies the third stage of adrenal fatigue, exhaustion. When cortisol and DHEA levels are persistently low, disease will eventually follow. The necessity of adequate quality sleep cannot be overemphasized for optimal health.

After this, T.M. got serious about getting more rest. His cortisol and DHEA levels came back to where they needed to be. His goals of more energy and increased muscle mass were achieved. More importantly, he avoided a potential life-changing health crisis. However, it took approximately one year before his adrenals fully recovered.

Chapter 8 References

1. Romanoff LP, Morris CW, Welch, P, Pincus G. Secretion rate of cortisol and daily excretion of tetrahydrocortisol, tetrahydrocortisol, or coralline (20 alpha and 20 beta). *J. Clin Endocrinol Metab* 1961, 21:1431.
2. Talbo, S. *The Cortisol Connection.* Alameda, CA: Hunter House Publications; 2007.
3. Tai PL. *8 Powerful Secrets of Anti-Aging.* Dearborn, MI: Health Secrets, USA; 2007.
4. Tai PL. *Clinical Nutrition.* Dearborn Heights, MI: Health Secrets, USA; pending publication.
5. Leaf C. *Switch on Your Brain.* Grand Rapids, MI: Baker Books; 2013.

Chapter 9: Aldosterone

Aldosterone is converted from progesterone through the intermediary of a mineralocorticoid, produced in the adrenal cortex. Although this book is focused primarily on the sex hormones, it is important to understand what aldosterone does in the body. Aberrations in aldosterone levels can occur when the adrenal glands are not functioning properly (adrenal fatigue). As we discussed in the Cortisol Chapter, ACTH (adrenocorticotrophic hormone) from the pituitary stimulates cortisol production. ACTH plays a small part in the production and secretion of aldosterone as well.

Aldosterone controls the fluid volume in the body, which is needed to help create blood pressure. Aldosterone increases volume pressure to push the blood into the brain when we stand up. Without this function, the fluid volume in the brain would drop when we stood up because of gravity. It also influences the fluid volume by inhibiting or enhancing potassium and sodium levels in the body. The balance of sodium and potassium not only helps to maintain appropriate fluid volumes, but also maintains the electricity in cells.

The major target of aldosterone is the distal tubules of the kidney. The three primary physiological effects of aldosterone are increased resorption of sodium, increased resorption of water with the consequential expression of extracellular fluid volume, and increased excretion of potassium. Therefore, when the adrenal cortex is under-functioning or there is adrenal fatigue, four physiological changes occur in the body: (1) The concentration of potassium in extracellular fluid becomes elevated; (2) the urinary excretion of sodium is higher while the concentration of sodium in the extracellular fluid decreases; (3) the volume of extracellular fluid and blood decreases; and (4) the heart begins to function poorly while cardiac output declines. These are fairly common complications in the elderly.

The four tissues target by aldosterone most are the distal tubules of the kidney, the saliva glands, the sweat glands, and the colon. Aldosterone stimulates the resorption of the sodium in the distal tubules of the kidneys, which increases fluid volume. Aldosterone also inhibits saliva and sweat production and the water resorption in the colon to increase fluid volume. Where aldosterone stimulates the resorption of sodium in the distal tubules, it is simultaneously stimulation the renal excretion of potassium. The more you excrete potassium the more sodium is retained and fluid volume is retained. Conversely, if you have too much fluid volume, you want to supplement or take in potassium and this will reduce fluid volume. The balance of sodium and potassium and, consequently, the fluid volume balance act like a perpetual seesaw in the body. To summarize, one of the life-threating physiological conditions we are most concerned about with aldosterone is when there is significant adrenal fatigue, which ultimately affects many heart functions, in particular cardiac output.

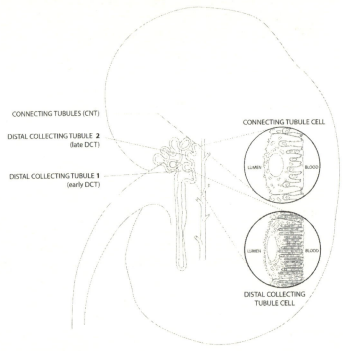

Chapter 9 Reference

1. Tai PL. *Clinical Nutrition*. Dearborn Heights, MI: Health Secrets USA; pending publication.

DHEA, *dehydroepiandrosterone*, is known as the father of all hormones. It represents the largest pool of hormones in the body. DHEA is converted from pregnenolone in the endoplasmic reticulum of the adrenal cortex where it is converted to either testosterone or estrogen through intermediaries. See diagram below.

The Hormone Pathways
DHEA

© Kelly Miller, DC NMD FASA FBAARM

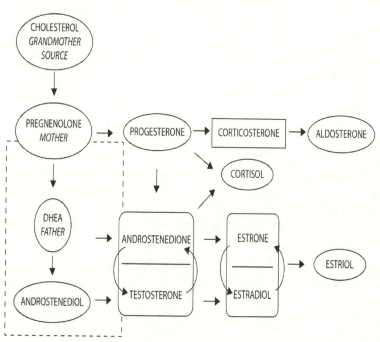

At age twenty-five, our DHEA levels are at their peak. After that age, we lose about two percent each year, depending on lifestyle and stress levels. At about age fifty, on average, we only produce about fifty percent of the amount we did at age twenty-five. By age seventy-five, most of us have negligible levels and are out of luck if we don't replenish by supplementation. Because DHEA affects almost every organ in the body, DHEA is also known as the *fountain of youth* hormone as it is thought by some to represent longevity potential.

DHEA affects almost every organ in the body. It is an anabolic (building) hormone that possesses the ability to heal and construct tissue. The many functions of DHEA include decreasing blood cholesterol, fatty deposits in the blood vessels, allergic reactions, and incidence of blood clots; improving bone growth, brain function, a sense of well-being, stress management, and cell repair; facilitating weight loss; supporting the immune system; and increasing the production of testosterone.[1,2] As the brain has five to ten times more DHEA than is in the blood plasma, it is vital to brain functions.

Symptoms of low levels of DHEA are depression, difficulty with handling stress, lack of stamina, moodiness, dry eyes, osteoporosis, memory loss, bone joint, and muscle pain. These symptoms—obesity, type 2 diabetes, depression, loss of sense of well being, cognitive dysfunction, loss of libido, erectile dysfunction, and osteoporosis—are also associated with low levels of DHEA.[1,2]

Chronic stress produces prolonged excessive amounts of cortisol and dominates the pathway from pregnenolone, inhibiting the conversion to DHEA. This is known as pregnenolone steal.[3] (See the pregnenolone steal chart in the chapter on cortisol.) As a consequence, chronic stress that causes excessive cortisol interferes with the production of DHEA and the anabolic physiology (healing, repair, and regrowth of new tissue) in the body. This is just another example that demonstrates that a single hormone excess or deficiency never exists in the body. Because of this phenomenon, physicians should never supplement a single hormone, such as testosterone or estradiol, without consideration of all the other hormones. Supplementation for multiple hormones is always required in an imbalanced hormonal system.

Some of the benefits of optimal levels of DHEA are increased muscle strength and lean mass; improved immune function, quality of life, sleep, feeling of wellness, sensitivity to insulin; decreased joint pain; lowered fatty triglycerides; and negated damaging effect of stress. [1-4] DHEA supplementation has positive effects for men suffering from declining muscle mass, increased body fat around the waist and middle of the body, libido reduction, fatigue, dry skin, energy loss, and strength loss. Supplementation has positive effects on women as an anti-depressant and anti-anxiety agent. It improves libido and skin thickness.[1-4]

Optimal levels of DHEA have also been found to reduce risk for breast, lung, colon, liver, skin, and lymphatic cancers.[5,6] DHEA concentration in the body is independently, and inversely, related to death from any cause and death from cardiovascular disease in men over age fifty.[1-3] In one study of 1700 men aging from forty to seventy, the men in the lowest quartile (25%) of reference range DHEA levels had the most ischemic heart disease. As with all hormones, optimal function occurs in the upper reference ranges. Optimal function occurs when all the hormones are balanced. If one hormone is deficient, other hormones will be deficient as well. As I have stated previously, it has been my experience that the best form of supplementation of DHEA is the transdermal application with liposome technology.

It has been well-established that a transdermal DHEA supplement is ten times more effective than oral pill form.[7-8] This *first pass* technology allows the hormone to be taken to the cell receptors via the capillaries where it will be readily used, leaving little, if any, to be sent on to the liver. This methodology spares the over-worked liver from having to produce *SHBG* (Sex Hormone Binding Globulin). Among its many benefits, transdermal DHEA supplementation has shown positive effects in slowing the progression of cardiovascular disease. It is also ant-aging, ant-obesity, and anti-diabetes.[9-12] DHEA supplementation has shown positive effects in slowing the progression of cardiovascular disease.

Take the DHEA self-assessment to help you determine if you may be experiencing a DHEA imbalance in your body

DHEA SELF-ASSESSMENT [1]
(Used with author's permission)

DHEA Deficiency	DHEA Excess
If supplementation has begun, increase dosage.	If supplementation has begun, decrease dosage.
Depression	Facial hair
Poor stress management	Oily skin
Lack of stamina	Acne, pimples
Moodiness	Bossiness
Dry eyes	Impatience, anger
Osteoporosis	Irritability, mood changer
Memory loss	Deepening voice
Bone, joint, muscle pain	

Chapter 10 References

1. Tai, PL. *8 Powerful Secrets to Anti-Aging*. Dearborn Heights, MI: Health Secrets USA; 2007.
2. Ahlgrimm, M. *The HRT Solution*. New York: Avery Pub; 1999.
3. Pregnenolone Steal, 2016. https://www.functionalmedicineuniversity.com/members/login.cfm?hpage=forum%2Fopenthread.cfm%3Fforum%3D15%26threadid%3D2420&cfmbbthreadid=2420. Accessed 04/01/2015
4. Lieberman, S. *The Real Vitamin and Mineral Book*. New York: Avery Pub; 1997.
5. Baulieu EE, Thomas G, Legrain S, et al. Dehydroeplandrosteron (DHEA), DHEA Sulfate and aging contributions of the DHEA age study to socio-biomedical issue. *Proceedings from the National Academy of Sciences USA*, 2000; 97(8) 4279-4284.
6. Schwartz A. Cancer prevention with DHEA. *Journal of Cellular Biochemistry*, 1998; 59(S22):210-212.
7. McCormick DL, Rao KV. Chemoprevention of hormone-dependent prostate cancer in wistar unilever rats. *The Journal of European Urology*, 1999; 35:464-467.
8. Labrie, C, Belanger. A., et al. High bioavailability of DHEA administered percutaneously in the rat. *Journal of Endocrinology*, 1996; 150:S107-118.
9. Hansen PA, Han DH, Nolte LA, Holloszy J.. DHEA protects against visceral obesity and muscle insulin resistance in rats fed a high-fat diet. *American Journal of Physiology*, 1997 Nov; 273 (5pt2): R1704-8.
10. Herrington DM. Dehydroepiandrosterone and coronary atherosclerosis. *Annals of New York Academy of Sciences*, 1995 Dec; 774:1271-80.
11. Morales AJ, Nolan JJ, Nelson JC, Yen SS. Effects of replacement dose of dehydroepiandrosterone in men and women of advancing age. *Journal of Clinical Endocrinology and Metabolism*, 1994 June; 78 (6): 1360.
12. Gordon GB, Bush DE, Weisman HF. Reduction of atherosclerosis by administration of

dehydroepiandrosterone. A study in the hypercholesterolemic New Zealand white rabbit with aortic intimal injury. *Journal of Clinical Investigations,* 1998 Aug; 82(2):712-20.

Testosterone is derived primarily from DHEA and secondarily from progesterone. Testosterone is produced primarily in the testes by men and in the adrenal cortex by women. See diagram below.

The Hormone Pathways
Testosterone

© Kelly Miller, DC NMD FASA FBAARM

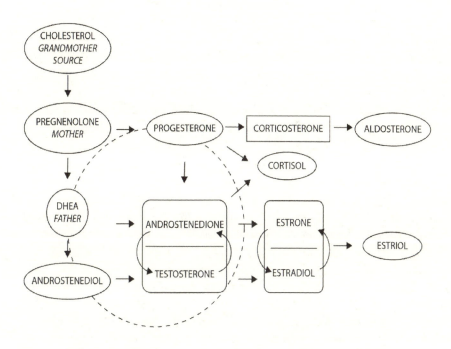

Testosterone is not just for men. It is just as vital for women. The cycle of reproduction of testosterone begins with the hypothalamus producing gonadotropic hormones that cause the anterior pituitary to produce *LH (luteinizing hormone)*, which has a direct effect on the testosterone production from the testes. Gonadotropic hormones from the hypothalamus also stimulate the production and secretion of FSH *(follicular stimulating hormone)*

from the pituitary, which is responsible for the production of sperm in the testes. LH (luteinizing hormone) and FSH (follicular stimulating hormone) affect the ovaries in a woman and initiate and control the menstrual cycle and ovulation.

As testosterone is produced, it is released into the bloodstream, creating a negative feedback system involving the hypothalamus and anterior pituitary. Receptor sites in the hypothalamus monitor the need for more testosterone production. When testosterone drops to a certain level in the blood, then the hypothalamus produces more gonadotrophic hormones that stimulate the anteriorly pituitary to produce and secrete more LH (luteinizing hormone), which, in turn, stimulates the testosterone production in the testes. Conversely, if testosterone levels rise to a certain point, the hypothalamus stops the production and secretion of the gonadotrophic hormone, which stops the anterior pituitary from producing and secreting LH. At this point, production of testosterone comes to a halt. Testosterone production occurs in two- to three-hour cycles throughout a twenty-four hour period, being the highest in the early morning.

Testosterone plays a role in many body functions. It affects muscle strength, size, and endurance because it affects the glucose utilization in the mitochondria of the cells. The thyroid hormone also influences the energy utilization within the mitochondria. A deficiency of either testosterone or thyroid hormone causes a lack of energy. Testosterone also affects bone growth development and strength while estrogen closes the epiphysis (end part of a long bone) of bones to end the growth cycle in puberty. Finally, testosterone affects the brain, social interactions, and libido and gives confidence.

Testosterone's effects are greatest on those tissues that contain the greatest amount of testosterone receptors. As I have emphasized in previous chapters, without proper functioning receptors, optimum cell activity cannot occur, even with high level of testosterone. The importance of proper functioning receptors is a critical concept for you to understand. The hormone level is only half of the equation. It is the optimum level of hormone coupled with proper functioning receptors that create optimum cell function and optimum health. Testosterone, DHEA, androstenedione, and DHT (*dehydrotestosterone*) are all considered androgenic (tissue building) hormones. Their relative values as androgens are one hundred percent for testosterone, five percent for DHEA, ten percent for

---

56

androstenedione, and three hundred percent for DHT.[1]

The free testosterone goes to the receptor site, is taken inside the cell, and is then converted to DHT, which is a three-times-more-powerful androgen than testosterone. From there, it is transported inside the nucleus of the cell. Besides the testes, the organ that has the most testosterone receptor sites is the heart. Optimum testosterone levels increase vasodilation, improve exercise tolerance, and improve angina threshold. Optimum testosterone levels also reduce visceral and body fat, maintain muscle and bone mass, memory, intelligence, and libido.

Hypothalamus-Pituitary-Gonads (HPG) Axis

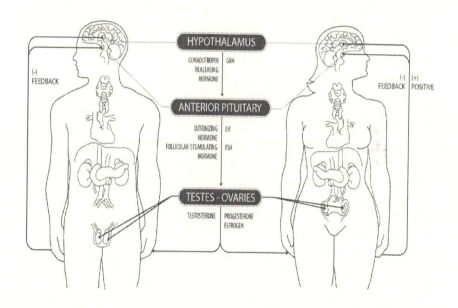

The most important hormone is free, not bound, but only about two percent of the total testosterone is free. Free testosterone denotes the hormone that is bio-available to bind with a testosterone receptor site in a cell. The other ninety-eight percent of testosterone found in the blood is bound with protein and cannot bind to a testosterone cell receptor site. The testosterone in the blood is bound with either SHBG, which accounts for sixty percent of the bound hormone, or albumin, which accounts for the other thirty-eight percent of the bound hormone. The SHBG molecule is large. In fact, it is so large that it will not go through the ducts that produce saliva. Consequently, the testosterone measured in the saliva is free, not bound. This is why saliva hormone testing is the most accurate measurement of only the testosterone that is bio-available to bind to a testosterone receptor site. Therefore, testosterone levels measured in the saliva are much more useful than blood serum testosterone levels in measuring testosterone.

Saliva reference range for testosterone levels for men should be 145-155 ng/dl. Reference range saliva testosterone levels for women should be 45-50 ng/dl. However, ideal levels are higher and are achieved with transdermal dosing.

While there is a difference of opinion on what is considered a low total testosterone level in the blood serum, the level of 350 ng/dl has been set as the lower limit by the Endocrine Society,[2] and the level of 300 ng/dl has been set by the International Society for the Study of Aging Males.[3] At either of these levels, men demonstrate *hypogonadism*, clinical under-functioning of the body to produce testosterone. At either level, a man is in deep trouble, in my opinion. Reference levels in most labs for serum total testosterone in men fall between 350-1150 pg/dl, and in women 10-55 pg/dl. However, ideal levels are higher and can be achieved with transdermal dosing.

You should always keep in mind that reference ranges are designed to keep eighty to ninety percent of the population within those parameters. Are any of us naïve enough to think that eighty to ninety percent of the American population is healthy? Numerous studies reflect that there is a huge difference in incidence of disease being in the lowest quartile (25%) of reference range vs. the upper quartile (25%). Healthier, more optimum, levels for men are 800-1150 ng/dl, or slightly higher, and 50-80 ng/dl for women.

Testosterone levels start declining in men at age twenty-five at the rate of approximately twenty percent each decade. This is one of the reasons it is so difficult for athletes in their mid-to-late thirties to compete against athletes in their lower twenties. There usually has been a significant loss in strength, endurance, and, most important, recovery by this time frame of ten to fifteen years. When a man reaches age fifty, he has lost on average fifty percent of his testosterone and is now in *andropause*, the male version of menopause in women. The physiological and biochemical changes that occur in men at this age are life threatening! Independent of all other of factors, a man's risk for heart attack doubles with a fifty percent reduction in testosterone levels. Andropause is additionally associated with a range of phenomenon: increased belly fat, decreased muscle mass and tone, decreased memory, decreased decision making, moodiness, irritability, fatigue, increased stiffness in the joints and muscles, loss of libido, decreased morning erections, decreased fullness of erections, decreased intensity of orgasm, and increased recovery time between orgasms.

Hypogonadism in men is a clinical syndrome that results from the failure of the testes to produce physiological levels of testosterone (below 300-340 ng/dl), and the normal amount of *spermatozoa* due to disruption of one or more levels of the HPG (hypothalamus-pituitary-gonad) axis. The HPG axis functions in a similar manner as the HPA (hypothalamus-pituitary-adrenal) axis discussed in prior chapters. It functions as a negative feedback system.

The HIM Study demonstrates what percentage of men had other concomitant conditions accompanying their hypogonadism and the risk factor involved in each condition. The following chart reveals how threatening these changes can be with men at least forty-five years of age with low testosterone/hypogonadism.[4] Low testosterone levels significantly increase the risk of occurrence of many diseases and illnesses.

Condition	% of Incidence	Odds
Obesity	52.6	2.38
Diabetes	50	2.09
Hypertension	47.3	1.84
Rheumatoid Arthritis	42	1.59
Hyperlipidemia	44.4	1.47
Osteoporosis	43.5	1.41
Asthma/COPD	41.3	1.40
Prostate Disease/Disorder	40.48	1.29
Chronic Pain	38.8	1.13
Headaches w/in 2 weeks	32.1	.81

The Massachusetts Male Aging Study, a large epidemiological study of American men over the last thirty years, demonstrates that the average testosterone levels in American men have been declining over the last three decades.[3] Why aren't men more aware of the signs and symptoms of low testosterone and the associated health risks? Why are doctors not screening men for this decline? A recent Harris Interactive poll survey of 522 men showed ninety-one percent of the men polled were not even aware of what symptoms were associated with low testosterone.[6] Because of this lack of data, I believe that every man and woman should get a saliva hormone test by the age forty.

Women also need testosterone to have a sense of well being. Women need testosterone to maintain muscular strength, especially in the upper body. Testosterone is responsible, in part, for a woman's libido and a woman's nipple and clitoral sensitivity. Testosterone is essential in women for body composition and bone density. Testosterone usually decreases in peri-menopausal and post-menopausal women. The aging woman often suffers from a *Relative Androgen Deficiency,* despite exhibiting normal reference ranges of testosterone.

The prevalence of many conditions—such as decreased cardiac output,[7] obesity,[7] type II diabetes,[7] *metabolic syndrome,* [7] AIDS,[8] hypertension,[7] hyperlipidemia,[7] erectile dysfunction,[9] coronary artery disease,[8] inflammation,[9] fracture from osteoporosis,[10-11] prostate cancer,[12] dementia,[13, 14] Alzheimer's,[13-15] and increased mortality—occurs in men from ages fifty to ninety-one, whose testosterone levels fall in the lowest quartile (25%) of the reference range.[8]

Testosterone levels are inversely related to central obesity, systolic blood pressure, and HgA1C (a test for diabetes). In one study, men who had levels over 564 ng/dl of testosterone in their blood had a forty-one percent less chance of dying compared to men with levels of 350 ng/dl of testosterone.[16] For every increase of 173 ng/dl of testosterone, the change of dying went down by fourteen percent. This means that a man with a testosterone level of 910 ng/dl would have a sixty-nine percent decreased risk of dying compared to the man with a testosterone level of 350 ng/dl.[17] This particular study was done evaluating *endogenous* testosterone levels in men vs. men with supplementing testosterone, demonstrating the benefits of supplementing bio-identical testosterone. In another study of eight hundred men over the age of fifty who were followed for eighteen years, there was a thirty-three percent increase in all deaths of those men in the bottom third of the reference range vs. men in the upper third of the reference range for testosterone levels.[13]

Fortunately, there is something you can do. There are a number of natural products that elevate testosterone levels including, but not limited to, *calcium fructoborate, Tribulus Terristrus, Eurycoma,* and *Panex Ginseng.*[14] A combination of these can help a fifty-year-old raise his testosterone levels close to fifty percent. Testosterone replacement therapy has been shown to decrease body and visceral fat, increase muscle mass, strength and endurance,[17, 20] increase bone density, improve cognitive function, decrease insulin resistance, improve lipid blood profiles, reduce depression,[21] and increase feelings of well-being.[22]

Contrary to many doctor's beliefs, testosterone replacement therapy has not been shown to increase prostate cancer, elevate *PSA* (prostate specific antigen) levels or increase the risk of prostate cancer from returning.[23] However, if a man has received testosterone suppressing medications for prostate cancer, he should not ever take supplemental testosterone.[24] In reviewing all the literature, it appears to be a myth that prostate cancer is perpetuated or caused by testosterone.[25] In fact, the research confirms that men with the lowest levels of testosterone appear to be at the greatest risk for developing prostate cancer. It also appears that men have a higher risk when their testosterone levels drop and estrogen levels elevate due to *aromatization* (conversion of testosterone to estrogen via the *aromatase* enzyme) after the age of fifty or sixty. What most men don't realize is that the average fifty-year-old male produces more estrogen than a menstruating twenty-year-old woman. This excess estrogen is what causes the prostate hypertrophy and prostate cancer[24,26] as the estrogen receptor sites in the prostate have been overstimulated.

There are two prestigious organization that have endorsed bio-identical testosterone supplementation: Life Extension and Harvard School of Medicine.[25] Life Extension recommends even higher levels of testosterone than Harvard School of Medicine. In the book, *Testosterone for Life,* Dr. Abraham Morgentaler, associate professor at Harvard School of Medicine, explains his favorable position regarding testosterone supplement in the aging male to reduce the many risks we have been discussing.[26] He discusses the fallacy of exogenous testosterone as a cause of prostate cancer in great detail. His research indicated an eighty-eight percent increased morbidity rate in men with low testosterone levels.

Testosterone levels are tested in one of three ways: through the blood, through the urine, or through the saliva. Remember that testosterone levels roller coaster up and down every two to three hours during a twenty-four hour period, fluctuating as much as eight hundred percent. It is highest in the morning. However, when evaluating testosterone from a blood draw, it is impossible to determine if your levels are in the peak or the valley of a cycle. The testosterone reading is merely a snapshot of twenty-four hour movie. I recommend never having your blood drawn in the afternoon to evaluate testosterone levels as, more likely than not, the reading will be low. Another problem with testing testosterone in the blood is that it is all bound to either SHBG or albumin. The fact is that all of this testosterone is inactive and on the way out of the body. In other words, your body cannot use any of this bound-hormone to activate the cell receptor sites.

A more accurate, though cumbersome, way to evaluate testosterone and the evaluation of other sex hormones is a twenty-four hour urine sample. This method requires you to collect all of your urine in a container during a twenty-four hour period, keep it refrigerated, and then get it to the lab. The third method of testing, saliva, is accurate especially when you collect five samples in three-hour increments during the day. Testing is achieved by the use of a simple straw, depositing a small amount of saliva through a straw into a plastic container. Saliva is stable for three to four weeks at room temperature. As noted earlier, saliva hormone testing only evaluates the free testosterone, the two percent that is unbound that can be used to activate the receptor site. I prefer saliva testing for my patients for all these reasons.

Once testosterone levels have been evaluated and found below optimum levels, there are a number of different ways to administer the hormone. The first option is to use a synthetic form of testosterone, which I never recommend to anyone because of increased risk for heart attack, strokes, and blood clots. What the so-called experts who promote synthetic testosterone don't tell you is that a FDA approved synthetic testosterone costs about $200/month vs. a compounded bio-identical testosterone that costs about $50/month. Moreover, synthetic testosterone is an extra-terrestrial molecule that is not designed for your body. Hormones work in a specific lock (receptor) / key (hormone) mechanism, and this synthetic key is not ideally suited for your lock. While it may open the door, it may damage the lock. Because synthetic hormones have to be altered from their original molecular structure in order to patent them, we are now seeing many class action suits against the synthetic form of testosterone because of the documented increased incidence of heart attack, stroke and blood clots after its usage. This is exactly what was discovered with women using synthetic estrogen. Unfortunately for women, it took almost seventy years before this hazard was exposed. I warned of the risk factors associated with synthetic testosterone in my newsletters and blogs back in 2013 even before the class action suits began.

The administration of bio-identical testosterone can be in oral (pill) form, injection form, surgically implanted pellet form, or in the form of transdermal patches or creams. There are several pros and cons of the different applications. The administration of oral testosterone can sometime alter taste buds or irritate the gums. Also absorption rates can vary among individuals and can result in too much testosterone being absorbed with the subsequent increased production of SHBG to compensate. The problem with a supra-physiological level (higher than body is capable of producing) is that the level is monitored by the hypothalamus, and the excess sets off an alert that sends a signal to the liver to produce the SHBG. The increased production of SHBG is indiscriminate about what hormone will be bound. As a result, all sex hormones become bound, lowering all hormone levels. This process also puts undue stress on a liver that is probably already over-worked.

Intramuscular injections can cause fluctuation in mood and libido as supra-physiological doses are given weekly, bi-monthly, or monthly, depending on the recommendations of the treating physician. These supra-physiological doses of testosterone can cause the activation of SHBG, and the injection can be painful. Some doctors may go to a two/week schedule to keep testosterone levels more in line with natural readings, but who wants to go to the doctor's office twice a week forever? Also, there is an increased risk for excessive *erythrocytosis,* a problem involving the red blood cells with injections.

Pellet implants are surgically inserted every two to three months. An incision has to be made. There is a possibility of

---

infection with all surgical procedures. Sometimes the body expels the pellets. If dosing is incorrect, the pellet has to be removed before the two to three month period is over. There also can be a problem with a steady dispersion of the hormone to the body. Finally, transdermal patches are an effective alternative, but can sometimes cause a skin reaction at the application site.

Seventy percent of the time, transdermal cream/gels are recommended by doctors. I prefer this methodology, coupled with liposome technology, as this ensures the best passage into the cell. Transdermal cream with liposome technology is also known as *first pass technology*. The capillary system takes the hormone to the receptor site in the cell where it binds and is used up before the hormone gets into the bloodstream to circulate to the liver. Therefore, very little if any, production of SHBG is triggered.

I want to emphasize that I believe no one should take testosterone without keeping the estradiol/estrone levels in check. As men age, they convert more testosterone to estrogen via the aromatase enzyme. Too high or too low levels of estrogen are detrimental to the health of men and women. As they age, there is a tendency to have a higher estrone levels. This increased production of estrogen not only increases the risk for prostate hypertrophy and cancer but increased cardiovascular risk for men. A recent study published in *The Journal of the American Medical Association (JAMA)* measured blood estradiol levels in 501 men with chronic heart failure. Men in the highest estradiol quartile were 133% were more likely to die than men in the healthy quartile. Men in the lowest quartile were 317% more likely to die compared to the healthy quintile group. The men in the healthiest quintile group had some estradiol level between 21.80 and 30.11 pg/ml.[23] Again this study shows a balance of hormone is important. The deficiency of testosterone and excess of estrogen is epidemic in aging men.

There are two patterns of testosterone deficiency in men. The first is characterized by non-specific reduction of testosterone production. There is normal or slightly elevated FSH/LH (follicular stimulating hormone/luteinizing hormone) that stimulate testosterone/sperm production respectively, and there are low estrone/estradiol levels. These are normal aging changes in some men. The other pattern of low testosterone is accompanied with high estrogen, normal or slightly low FSH/LH, *Syndrome X, NIDDM* (non-insulin dependent diabetes mellitus), and obesity.

One of the ways that this problem can be addressed is with the administration of natural aromatase inhibitors. There are a number of natural aromatase inhibitors and/or estrogen detoxifiers that help give protection to the prostate in men and breast, uterus, and ovaries in women. These nutrients include, but are not limited to, Vitamin C, *quercetin*,[24] *nettles*,[25,26] *indole -3- carbinol*, (1-3-C), diindolylmethane (DIM), resveratral, chrysin,[30] and *peperine extract*.[31]

You should keep in mind that a single hormone deficiency never exists. This is true for testosterone as well. If there is a testosterone deficiency, there is a concomitant deficiency in both pregnenolone and DHEA as well because these two hormones are in the pathway of production of testosterone.[32] All hormones, including testosterone, have to be *hydroxylated, methylated,* or *sulfated* to be made water soluble so that they can be excreted from the body through sweat, urine, or feces. Some of these metabolites are carcinogenic in the hydroxylated form, for example, C-4 hydroxyestrone and especially C-16 alpha-hydroxyestrone. These metabolites are a potential problem for both men and women. This is discussed in greater detail in the next chapter on estrogen.

The Case of Too Much Testosterone

The following case study is about a fifty-three-year-old male who was being seen by another physician, but had come to me for another opinion and alternative care. This case demonstrates multiple points I have made in this book. S.C. was a very enthusiastic individual with great energy when he had it. He had a history of attention deficit and had been medicated for it when he was younger. However, he had been off of this medication for years until recently. To his previous physician's credit, he had done an extensive and fairly thorough work-up on this patient. Being a good doctor has two parts. The first part is being able to correctly diagnose the problem(s) and the second part is to be able to recommend a program that will resolve the issue(s). I will give the other physician an "A" for the first part, but a "C-" on the recommendations.

S.C. had a history of sleep apnea, type II diabetes, and elevated cholesterol and triglycerides, which had improved but not resolved. He was overweight and reported that he had constipation.

and fluctuating energy levels that were worse in the afternoon. He also told me he had low testosterone and had the *E4/E4* gene variant that increases the risk for cardiovascular disease and Alzheimer's disease. He was a classic case of Metabolic Syndrome or Syndrome X. He brought in his last two test results for his sex hormones and thyroid hormones, an extended metabolic and cardiovascular risk panel, and a *C.B.C.* (complete white and red blood cell count).

The test results indicated that he had extremely elevated triglycerides, blood glucose, *homocysteine* (a marker for increased risk of heart attack and even more so for a stroke), testosterone, and estradiol. He had been prescribed too high a dose of testosterone and was converting much of it into estrogen. Elevated estradiol levels increase the risk of a heart attack. The test results also indicated he had a *B pattern* in his LDLs, which is the result of a genetic trait. This means he had too many of the very small, sticky kind of lipoproteins carrying his cholesterol. He also had the E4/E4 gene variant that is associated with decreased efficiency in getting rid of *beta-amyloid* in the brain: Alzheimer's disease is marked by beta-amyloid deposits in the brain. His HDL (good cholesterol, larger lipoproteins carrying the cholesterol) levels were very low and were lower than the previous test. In addition, his thyroid hormone levels were in the lower quartile (25%) of reference range. I had the patient take his basal body temperature readings, and they averaged 96.3 F, about 2 degrees below the normal temperature of 98.6 F.

The big picture on this patient was that his elevated blood sugars and insulin resistance were the primary aggravating factors for causing his sex hormone deficiencies and for increasing his negative *epigenetic expression* of his B pattern LDLs and E4/E4 genetic variants. Although this patient could benefit from sex hormone therapy, fixing his blood sugar/insulin problems were key to get at the root cause of much of his multiple metabolic dysfunctions and to help accomplish weight loss and correction of his metabolism. His thyroid and adrenal glands functions were subpar. Adrenaline/cortisol and thyroid hormones are necessary for *every* cell's function. The function of the adrenals and thyroid are critical to the production of the sex hormones.

Recommendation for this patient by his prior physician included oral testosterone without pregnenolone or DHEA, an adrenal supplement, and an oral B12 supplement. Unfortunately, it is not wise to give testosterone without pregnenolone and DHEA support. The level of testosterone was too high, which caused the patient's symptoms of attention deficit/hyperactivity to increase, causing him to have to go back on prescription medications. He had already demonstrated elevated estradiol levels when his testosterone levels were low in initial evaluation by the other physician, indicating he was converting most of his testosterone to estradiol. As his testosterone level increased so did his estradiol level, putting him at higher risk for cardiovascular event. Men exhibiting high levels of estradiol/estrone should be placed on natural aromatase inhibitors to discourage the conversion from testosterone to estradiol and androstenedione to estrone. While his fasting glucose, insulin and total cholesterol levels were mildly improved, his triglycerides remained over 350 mg/dl (normal under 150 mg/dl) and his HDL was down to 29 mg/dl (ideal > 55 mg/dl in men), his B pattern of LDLs remained the same, and his cortisol levels remained low.

During my initial consultation with S.C. it was apparent that his *ADHD* was out of control, causing erratic thinking and behaviors that resulted in poor choices sometimes. He often worked extended hours during the day into the evening without eating. Then he went home and ate continually for two hours from 8-10 PM. Many times he did not go to bed until after midnight. Something had to change in his daily activities for him to get well. As he was a spirit-filled man, I began by appealing to him that he had a responsibility to take better care of his temple.

> Beloved, I pray that you may prosper in all things and be in health, just as your soul prospers. *3 John 2.*
> Now may the God of peace Himself sanctify you completely; and may your whole spirit, soul, and body be preserved blameless at the coming of our Lord Jesus Christ. *I Thessalonians 5:23.*

This approach registered with him.

We began by starting him on a ten-day program of eating only baked and broiled meats, vegetables, and berries and a vegetable-based protein shake, adding some flaxseed and the berries to it with some blood sugar regulating supplements, including *gymnema* (herb to increase pancreatic beta cell function that produces insulin), chromium, alpha lipoic acid, and more. He also agreed to prepare his meals at his office as he had a kitchen there, not to eat after 8 PM, and get to bed by 10 PM. Not sleeping adequately damages the adrenal glands by adversely effecting cortisol levels, which increases blood sugar regulating problems. As you may recall, the adrenal glands repair from 10 PM to 4 AM.

By the end of ten days, S.C. had lost twelve pounds and reported his energy was much better. His appearance was much improved with less darkening around his eyes, and his forehead had a nice pink color to it. After this initial ten-day period designed to help break his bad daily routine and improve his sugar/insulin metabolism, he was placed on a medical food product to help better regulate the peaks and valleys of his blood sugars and a blend of South American grasses to help balance his *neurotransmitters (dopamine, serotonin, GABA)* for his ADHD.

During this time he was given a saliva hormone test to better assess free hormone levels. Saliva hormone testing revealed low levels of DHEA and cortisol and elevated levels of estradiol and estrone. Based on these results and his symptoms, he was placed on transdermal pregnenolone, DHEA, *Max Andro* (a product to increase endogenous testosterone production by fifty percent), and natural aromatase inhibitors to discourage to the conversion of testosterone to estradiol, appropriate adrenal and thyroid nutraceutical support, a time released niacin to increase HDL, and a sublingual B vitamin with liposome technology to better support the methylation phase of estrogen detoxification and prevention of excess homocysteine. (See Estrogen chapter for more details.)

S.C. discontinued his oral testosterone, and within two weeks discontinued his prescription medication for ADHD. This patient continued to lose weight over the next three months for an additional thirty pounds. At the end of this three-month period, his fasting glucose levels were at 90, and his insulin levels were at 12 ulU/mL (optimum under 14ulU/mL), down from 20.3 ulU/mL. His HDL level was at 50 mg/dl (ideal>55 mg/dl), up from 29 mg/dl, homocysteine level was at 4.3 umol/L (ideal under 3 umol/L), down from 8.3 umol/L, and triglycerides were at 155 mg/dl (ideal 70-110 mg/dl, down from 322 mg/dl. His DHEA, testosterone levels were optimum, and his estradiol and estrone levels were ideal. His cortisol levels were improved. I informed him that it might take another three to nine months to get his cortisol levels ideal. The patient reported he was able to focus much better and was much more productive at work. He reported his energy was more even throughout the day, he was sleeping better, and his endurance during workouts was vastly improved as was his love life. I recommended that he keep his carbohydrate in-take to less than fifty percent of total caloric intake and have at least thirty percent fat in his daily intake.

As you may recall in my previous discussions, I stated that it is always important to ask the question—Why is this individual's hormone levels low? His testosterone levels were initially low at 300 pg/ml (reference range 400-1150 pg/ml). This was due to the following reasons: age, low thyroid function, elevated blood sugars/insulin, being overweight, and having poor eating habits and sleeping patterns. These root causes needed to be addressed for long-term health benefits for this patient. Although he did benefit from testosterone supplementation, supporting this hormone only was not a good solution. Testosterone supplementation should always be supported with pregnenolone and DHEA supplementation. As you may remember from the sex hormone pathway chart in Chapter 1, testosterone is converted from either DHEA or progesterone, both hormones coming from the conversion of pregnenolone. You will recall that a single hormone deficiency does not exist in the body.

Also, the adrenals and the thyroid must be balanced for the sex hormones to be balanced. (See the chart in Chapter 1.) Balanced cortisol produced from the adrenals is necessary for the cells that produce the sex hormones to work, and the thyroid hormones are necessary to determine the rate of function. Moreover, low thyroid function and high sugar levels increase LDL cholesterol and triglycerides. Improving blood sugars/insulin and thyroid function was critical to normalizing this patient's lipid profile, metabolism, all the sex hormones, not just testosterone, and reducing his risk for cardiovascular incidents and Alzheimer's.

Take this self-assessment to help determine if you are suffering from an imbalance in testosterone levels in your body.

Note Vi

TESTOSTERONE SELF-ASSESSMENT [1]
(Used with permission of the author)

Testosterones Deficiency

If supplementation has already been taken, increase dosage.

Flabby, weak muscles ✓
Low self-esteem
Loss of muscle mass ✓
Lack of confidence ✓
Mental fog ?⤵
Decreased libido ✓
Lack of orgasm or sex drive ✓
Depression
Thinning hair ✓

Fatigue ✓
Dry skin, thin skin lacking ·
elasticity · ✓ *yes*

Testosterone Excess

If supplementation has already been taken, decrease dosage.

Too aggressive
Bossiness, anxiety, agitation
Oily facial skin
Over confidence
Acne eruptions
Increased facial hair
Constant anger
Decreased HDL
Irregular menstrual cycles in women

Chapter 11 References

1. Tai, PL. *8 Powerful Secrets to Anti-Aging.* Dearborn Heights, MI: Health Secrets, USA: 2007.
2. Bhasin S, Cunningham GR, Hayes FS, et al. Testosterone Therapy in Adult Men with Androgen Deficiency Syndrome: An Endocrine Society Clinical Practice guidelines. *Journal of Clinical Endocrinology& Metabolism* 2010, Vol. 95(6):2536-2559.
3. Lunenfield B, Mskhalaya G, Zitzmann M, et al. Recommendations on the diagnosis, treatment, and monitoring of hypogonadal men. *The Aging Male.* **http://informahealthcare.com/tam**. ISSN: 1368-3538 (print). 1473-0790 (electronic).
4. Mulligan T, Frick MF, Zuraw QC, Stenhagen A, McWhirter C. Prevalence of hypogonadism in males aged at least 45 years: the HIM study. *Int. J. Clin. Pract.* 2006 Jul; 60(7):762-769.
5. O'Donnel AB, Araujo AB, McKinley JB. The health of normally aging men: The Massachusetts Male Aging Study (1987-2004). *Exp. Gerontol.* 2004 Jul;39(7):975-984.
6. "Low Testosterone: Man's Condition in the Shadows." Washington, April 18, 2006 /PRNewswire via COMTEX/
7. Laaksonen DE, Niskanen L, Punnonen K. Testosterone and sex hormone-binding globulin predict the metabolic syndrome and diabetes in middle-aged men. *Diabetic Care* 2004. 27(5):1036-1041.
8. Haring R, Volzke H, Stzveling A, et al. Low serum testosterone levels are associated with increased risk of mortality in a population-based cohort of men aged 20-79. *Eur. Heart Journal.* DOI: **http://dx.doi.org/10.1093/eurheartj/ehq009** First published online: 17 February 2010.
9. Caretta N, et al. Erectile dysfunction in aging men. Testosterones role in therapeutic protocols. J *Endocrinol Invest* 2005;28(11 Supp Proc)

10. Benito M. Effect of testosterone replacement on trabecular architecture in hypogonadal men. *J Bone Miner Res.* 2005:30(10):1785-9.
11. Amery, J.K. Testosterone & Changes in Bone Mineral Density. *J Clinical Endocrinol Metab* 2004; 89:503-510.
12. Schatzl G, Madersbacher S, Thurridi T, et al. High-grade prostate cancer is associated with low serum testosterone level. *The Prostate*, Volume 47, Issue 1, pages 52-58. 1 April 2001.
13. Rosario ER, Chang L, Stanczyk FZ, Pike CJ. Age related testosterone depletion and the development of Alzheimer's disease. *JAMA* September 22/29, 2004, Vol. 292, No. 12.
14. Tan RS, Pu SJ. A pilot study on the effects of testosterone on hypogonadal aging male patients with Alzheimer's disease. *The Aging Male*, Volume 6, Issue 1, 2003. DOI: 10.1080/tam.6.1.13.17
15. Gouras GK, Xu H, Gross R, et al. Testosterone reduces neuronal secretion of Alzheimer's beta –amyloid peptides. *Proc Nat'l Acad Sci USA* 2000 Feb1; 97(3):1202-5.
16. Svartberg J, Agledahl I, Figenschau Y, et al. Testosterone treatment in elderly men with subnormal testosterone levels improves body composition and BMD in the hip. *Int J Impot Res* 2008 Jul-Aug; 20(4):378-87.
17. Bhasin S, et al. Proof of the effect of testosterone on the skeletal muscle. *Am J Physiol Endocrino.* 2001.
18. Laughlin GA, Barret-Connor E, Bergstrom J. Low serum testosterone and mortality in older men. *J Clin Endocrinol Metab* 2008 Jan;93(1):68-75. Epub 2007 Oct. 2.
19. Adimoelja, A. Phytochemicals in the breakthrough of traditional herbs in the management of sexual dysfunction. *Int J Androl* 2000:23 Suppl 2:82-4.
20. Kenny AM, Kleppinger A, Annus A, et al. Effects of transdermal testosterone on bone and muscle in older men with low bioavailable testosterone, low bone mass, and physical frailty. *J Am Geriatr Soc* 210 Jun; 58(6):1134-43.

21. Carnahan RM, Perry PJ. Depression in aging men: the role of testosterone. *Drugs Aging* 2004; 21(6):361-76.
22. Morley JE, Testosterone and behavior. *Clin Geriatr Med* 2003 Aug;19(3):605-16. Review PMID: 14567011.
23. Marks LS, Mazer NA, Mostaghel E, et al. Effect of testosterone replacement therapy on prostate tissue in men with late-onset hypogonadism: a randomized controlled trail. *JAMA* 2006 Nov 15; 296(19):2351-61.
24. Roddam AW, Allen Ne, Appleby P, Key TJ. Endogenous sex hormones and prostate cancer: A collaborative analysis of 18 prospective studies. *J Natl Cancer Inst* 2008 Feb 6; 100(3):170-183.
25. Life Extension. *Male reproductive male hormone restoration.* http://www.lef.org/Protocols/Male-Reroductive-male-Hormone-Restoration/Page-01: 2016. Accessed 5/15/2016.
26. Morgentaler A, *Testosterone for Life: Recharging Your Vitality, Sex Drive, Muscle Mass, and Overall Health*, Amazon.com/books 2008.
27. Jankoska EA, Rozentryt P, Ponikowska B, et al. Circulating Estradiol and Mortality in Men with Systolic Heart Failure. *JAMA* 2009; 301(18);1892-1901.
28. Khan SI, Zhao J, Khai A, et al. Potential utility of natural products as regulation of breast –causing aromatase promotion. *Reprod Biol Endocrinol* 2001 Jun21;9:91.
29. Gannser D, Spiteller G. Aromatase inhibition from urtica dioitca roots. *Planta Med* 1995 Apr; 6192): 138-140.
30. Vonpoppel GFO. Brassica vegetables and cancer prevention. *Adv Exp Med Bio* 1999
31. Terry P. Brassica vegetables and breast cancer risk. *JAMA* 2000.
32. Bradlow HL. Indole-3-Carbinol as a chemoprotective agent in breast and prostate cancer. *In Vivo* 2008 Jul-Aug; 22(4): 44-5.
33. Sinha D, Saskar N, Biswar J, Bishayee A. Resveratrol for breast cancer prevention and treatment: Pre-clinical

evidence and molecular mechanisms. *Semin Cancer Biol* 2016 Jan 13. PMID: 26774195

34. Moon YJ, Wang X, Morris ME. Dietary flavonoids: effects on xenobiotic and carcinogenic metabolism. *Toxicol in Vitro* 2006 Mar; 20(20: 187-210.

35. Walle T, Otake Y, Brubaker JA, Walle UK, Halishka PV. Disposition and metabolism of the flavonoid chrysin in normal volunteers. *J Clin Pharmacol* 2001 Feb; 51(20; 143-6.

36. Tai PL. *Encyclopedia of Natural Products*, Ann Arbor, MI: BARM PMA Publishers: 2015.

Chapter 12: Estrogen

Estrogen is a group of compounds including estrone (E1), estradiol (E2), and estriol (E3). It is found in both women and men, but in much larger amounts in younger women than younger men. However, the average fifty-year-old man produces more estrogen in his body than a twenty-year-old menstruating woman.[1] On the other hand, the average twenty-year-old woman produces more testosterone than a sixty-year-old man.

Estrogen, like progesterone, is controlled by not only a negative feedback system but also a positive feedback system to the hypothalamus and pituitary. Refer to the H-P-G illustrations in Chapter 7 on progesterone and testosterone. Estradiol is converted from testosterone, and estrone is converted from androstenedione. (See the illustration below.)

The Hormone Pathways
Estrogen

© Kelly Miller, DC NMD FASA FBAARM

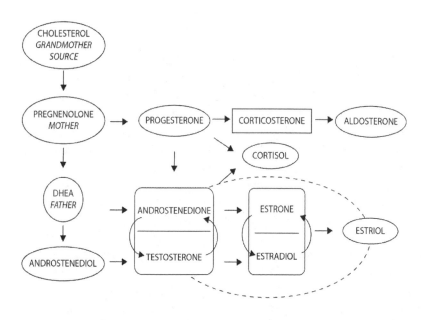

The production of estrogen occurs mostly in the *corpus luteum* (a hormone producing structure) of the ovum by the developing egg follicles. The placenta also produces it during pregnancy and, in lesser amounts, the liver, adrenal glands, and breasts produce it.[1] The ovaries as well as body fat produce estrone (E1). In fact, the more body fat one has the more estrone is produced. This is true for both women and men. Estrone is converted to estrone sulfate, which is a water-soluble reservoir that can be converted back to estrone as needed. Estrone levels are very relevant to health and disease states as excess increases the risk for cardiovascular disease and breast and prostate cancers.

Estradiol (E2) or 17B estradiol is the predominant sex hormone in women during their childbirth years. Estradiol exists in a large hormone pool with estrone (E1). Estradiol and estrone interchange as needed. Males also produce estradiol as an active metabolic product of testosterone. Estradiol represents the major form of estrogen in humans. As such, it has a major impact on reproduction, sexual functioning, and on many organs including the bones. Estradiol synthesis is derived from cholesterol via the delta-5 pathway or the delta-6 pathway, both crucial enzymes in the breakdown of polyunsaturated fatty acids. Androstenedione is the key intermediary. Part of androstenedione is converted to testosterone and part to estrone. In fact, testosterone undergoes conversion to estradiol by an enzyme called aromatase.

The third and probably least understood form of estrogen is estriol (E3). It is important in maintaining pregnancy, as levels increase one thousand percent as do progesterone levels during pregnancy. It is a benign and protective form of estrogen, meaning it does not have *carcinogenic metabolites* (by-products of metabolism) like estrone. Estriol is the end of the line for the cascade of all the hormones. The largest estriol (E3) production is during pregnancy. Estriol levels do not change much from premenopausal to postmenopausal. It is the smallest pool of estrogen and is protective of the breast, uterus, and ovaries. It is only found in minute amounts in men and is not considered to be important in men's health.

Some of the most important functions or roles of estrogen are that it increases metabolic rate, blood flow, reasoning and new ideas, water content of the skin, HDL (good cholesterol) by ten to fifteen percent concentration, and sexual interest. Estrogen decreases the plaquing in the arteries, blood pressure, and LDL (bad cholesterol) and prevents oxidation, Lipoprotein A (an inherited risk factor for cardiovascular disease), wrinkles, and risk of colon cancer. Estrogen helps to prevent muscle damage and maintains muscles, deep sleep, maintain memory, motor skills, and maintains bone mass. Estrogen contributes to the development of secondary sex characteristics, which include the breasts, the widened pelvis, and increased amounts of body fat in the buttocks, defining a difference between women and men.

The three compounds—estrone, estradiol, and estriol—are seen at work during the reproductive or follicular phase, which begins with the first menstruation and ends with menopause. During this time, estradiol is the dominant estrogen. Estradiol is converted from testosterone. The properties of estrogen are many and varied: It creates the *endometrium* (inner lining of the uterus) and sexual development at puberty, regulates menstrual cycle, moistens vaginal tissue, slows bone loss, and generally helps to prevent aging, increases sensitivity of progesterone receptors, and adds moisture to the skin. It actually affects more than three hundred tissues in the body, including the reduction of the incidence of heart attacks, mood elevation, lowering LDL, while increasing HDL, and decreasing lipoprotein A and homocysteine. Estrogen also affects every neurotransmitter in the brain including serotonin, *dopamine*, and *GABA*. It affects brain function for memory and motivation needed for verbal memory and to learn new concepts and reasoning and fine motor skills.

A significant reduction in estrogen occurs after menopause. The reduction in estrogen leads to vaginal dryness and shrinkage, memory problems, hot flashes, night sweats, irritability, and decrease in bone density. These negative symptoms can be negated with estradiol/estriol bio-identical supplementation. Estradiol affects bone growth, liver function, and brain function. Without it, there is no epiphyseal closure in our bones. Generally, tall and *eunuchoid* (having reduced or indeterminate sexual characteristics) women have a later onset of puberty, often due to high levels of melatonin, which delays the onset of puberty. Estradiol is what creates the protein matrix in the bone, and its loss can cause early osteopenia and osteoporosis.[2,3]

Estradiol has complex functions and affects the liver. Excess estradiol can lead to *cholestasis* (where the liver does not produce enough bile to digest fats). Estradiol affects the production of protein in the liver that is necessary to activate nitric oxide production, including lipoprotein A (a LDL that sticks to the arteries and increases heart attack by three hundred percent), and the protein responsible for blood clotting.

Estradiol affects many functions in the brain. It protects the nervous system from free radicals, acting as powerful anti-oxidant. Via estradiol, the ovaries are linked to the hypothalamus-pituitary through both a positive and negative feedback system that the gonadotropin hormones regulate. Estradiol regulates serotonin, dopamine, and GABA. Without adequate levels, depression can occur. When estradiol levels are not stable, it can lead to postpartum depression and *peri menopause* and menopause depression.[4-6]

During menopause, estriol controls hot flashes, insomnia, and vaginal dryness and shrinkage, and can be used as replacement therapy for these symptoms.[7-9] Estriol helps maintain the GI tract for the growth of good bacteria and reduces pathogenic bacteria. Estriol helps restore the normal PH of the vagina, which prevents urinary tract infections. It reverses atrophy of the vagina and thickens and moisturizes the vaginal lining.[10-12]

Estrogen also plays a role in the health of men. Testosterone is produced in the *Leydig cells* of the testicles. The testosterone is then carried to the tissues having estrogen receptor cells, where the conversion, via the aromatase enzyme, from testosterone to estradiol occurs. This aromatization occurs within the receptor cell itself. This local cellular aromatization was not discovered until the work of Dr. Sharpe in 1998. This local transference of testosterone into estradiol at the cellular level changes the way we think of estrogen-related cancers of the breast, uterus and ovaries.[13] In the past, it was thought that estrogen was brought to the receptor of the cell only through the bloodstream. Estrogen can also come from the body fat in men.

The hypothalamus has a high concentration of both alpha and beta estrogen receptors. These high levels of estrogen and aromatase receptors in the brain control a man's sexuality, his libido, and his erectile function. The brain is actually the largest sexual organ in the body, influencing many of the physical characteristics of sex. How does estrogen help with erectile dysfunction? Estrogen stimulates the production of nitric oxide that causes the vasodilatation (blood engorgement) in the pelvic and penile arteries and the sexuality centers in the brain. It is the estradiol that is necessary to activate the nitric oxide production.[14]

Estradiol is also necessary to the pro-inflammatory activity involved in vascular plaquing, such as *iNOS, MMPS, IL-6,* and *COX2* (all inflammatory markers). This is why men's cardiovascular risk increases if estradiol levels are too low (not enough nitric oxide), or too high (too much inflammation). It is interesting to note that too low of estradiol levels in men increases cardiovascular risk more than excess estradiol.

Estrogen alpha receptors and beta receptors are what actually provide the brain function of sexuality, the modulation of hormone secretion from the pituitary, the bone growth mineralization, epiphyseal (bone) closures, inhibition of bone resorption, the cardio-protective protection changes that increase HDL, lower LDL, increase vasodilation, the fat depositions, and fat utilization for energy, and the widespread effect on genital tissues and testicular function. There is aromatase activity (the conversion of testosterone to estradiol) in all these tissues. This means that these tissues are not dependent upon the circulating estradiol hormones in the blood.

In aromatization deficiency syndrome, the male *phenotype* features are preserved, but because of the lack of estradiol feedback the testes enlarge. Testosterone levels are two to three hundred percent above normal with very low estradiol levels. Erectile function is preserved, but the libido is low or absent. Reduced ossification occurs. Osteopenia or osteoporosis can occur like in a post-menopausal woman. It can cause a lack of epiphyseal closure, causing a taller status. There is increased atherosclerosis and calcification in the arteries because of the absence of estradiol protection.[15]

Low levels of estradiol affect other areas of health as well. Syndrome X or Metabolic Syndrome is known for the characteristics of increased LDL, increased triglycerides, low HDL2, *hyperinsulinism*, insulin resistance, early onset diabetes, obesity, and risk of hypertension. All these changes move toward normal with estradiol treatment, including the regression of carotid *atheromas* (accumulation of degenerative material in the arteries).[16]

Evaluating hormone levels in the blood, saliva, or urine only gives the doctor half of the information he or she needs regarding hormone function. The other half of the information is in the cell receptors that need the hormone. When the patient has classic symptoms of under function and normal reference ranges of hormone, receptor resistance should be suspected. It takes an astute doctor to recognize this.

Estrogen alpha-receptor *polymorphisms* or gene variants can occur. It is the alpha unit that first binds with the hormone and the beta unit that takes the hormone inside the cell. This particular alpha gene variant causes high estrogen levels. The phenotype appears normal. This means that the outside appearance of the man appears normal. However, this causes the same pathologies as aromatase deficiency syndrome, causing increased *atherogenesis* (causing degenerative material in the arteries) and other syndrome changes. Estradiol supplementation improves the health of the patient with estrogen alpha receptor polymorphism. Without the estradiol supplementation, the patient has increased cardiovascular risk and early onset of disease.[16,17]

Men can also have other problems with estrogen. There are some men who have an increase in aromatase because of their genetics. These individuals demonstrate gynecomastia at a young age. There is also an acquired estrogen dominance brought on by mid-life obesity and Syndrome X. These men exhibit poor response to testosterone supplementation as their levels of estrogen rise from aromatization. These men benefit from aromatase inhibitors. As men get older, they produce more estrone from androstenedione instead of testosterone in the adrenals and from body fat. Supplementation of *CoQ10, alpha lipoic acid, Vitamin E,* and zinc helps to facilitate the conversion of androstenedione to testosterone instead of estrone.[17]

Levels of estrogen are also important in the function of insulin production, just as they are in determining cardiovascular risk. Too much or not enough estradiol increases insulin resistance, just as it increases cardiovascular risk. Everything in nature is about balance. The higher estradiol and the lower testosterone are the more obese a person is and the higher the B.M.I index.[18]

Lower serum testosterone levels are seen with low SHBG (Sex Hormone Binding Globulin) normal free testosterone and higher estradiol and estrone levels with normal FSH/LH in obese men. Estradiol and estrone levels are proportionate to body fat. The greater the body fat, the higher the estrogen level. Other markers of estrogen excess are evident as signs of feminization, such as roundness of the belly, hips, and thighs and gynecomastia. In conclusion, if defective estrogen receptors are present, decreased testosterone is present as there is an increased clearance of

---

testosterone and occurrence of an elevated production of estrogen.[19]

There are two genetic variants of estrogen involving the 17 Beta HSD enzyme. If there is an increase in that particular enzyme, there is an increased aromatase activity causing the conversion of testosterone to estradiol. If there is a decrease of this enzyme, androstenedione is then converted to testosterone instead of estrone.[20]

Some types of coronary artery disease pathophysiology are influenced by estrogen. Coronary artery disease is marked by plaguing. There are two types of plaquing, one with calcification and one with soft plaquing. Coronary calcification is a highly significant factor in coronary artery disease, plaque, cerebrovascular events (strokes), and mortality. There is a poor association between this type of plaque and cholesterol and triglycerides and with traditional risk factors. This type of plaquing has a high correlation with steroid hormones, such as parathyroid hormone, estrogen, and testosterone.[21] Conversely, it is the soft plaque that is associated with the accumulation of VLDLs (very small sticky LDLs) and *sudden death* from the eruption of the soft plaque and *foam cells* (white blood cells called macrophages that are fat-laden). [22]This is the type of heart attack that instantly kills an individual.

Estrogen and Aging, Detoxification of Estrogen, and Genetic Variations

Mainstream Western medicine is based on the concept that we should look at *normal* people to determine different needs for vitamin, mineral, and antioxidant intake. This concept originated from Rogers Williams in 1956.[23] We now know there are several different types of *normal.* We have confirmation through genetic testing that there are many genetic variances among individuals that affect the way they absorb, use or react to certain nutrients or drugs. Moreover, this concept of variance among individuals is not new as the differences among individuals have been discussed in *Ayurvedic Medicine,*[24] *Chinese Traditional Medicine,*[25] and ancient Greek medicine.[26] These differences and influences have been taken into consideration in the diagnosis and treatment of individuals for thousands of years.

Science has just recently revalidated what was taken for granted long ago. Science has shown that different individuals have varying amounts of some receptors in their bodies that influence the

81

dosing of a particular nutrient or drug. Likewise, dosing should vary for these differences, such as different sized individuals, different types of metabolisms, different builds, acute vs. chronic conditions, and mild vs. severe conditions. This is true for hormone supplementation therapy as well. Dosing must be individualized based on the needs of the patients. For example, a large muscled hairy male may require more DHEA and testosterone than a slender, less hairy male. A woman with a more rounded figure with larger breast, hips, and buttocks will need more estrogen than a "twiggy" type woman.

Original synthetic hormones were called *triests* because they combined all three estrogens: estrone (E1), estradiol (E2), and estriol (E3). Because the estrone metabolites, such as 16-alpha-hydroxyestrone, can be very carcinogenic, physicians have stopped using estrone in formulations. Instead, physicians have opted for *Biest* formulations containing only estradiol and estriol. Estrone is closely related to our body mass index, overall insulin levels, and insulin receptors. Estradiol is the most potent form of estrogen, being twelve times more powerful than estrone, and eighty times more powerful than estriol. High levels of estradiol are associated with premenstrual syndrome, ovarian cysts, uterine fibroids, endometrial dysplasia, and increased risk for breast cancer. Most women suffering from P.M.S. have estradiol levels that are too high relative to their progesterone levels. Estriol is the smallest and weakest fraction of estrogen. Estriol is not carcinogenic and, in fact, demonstrates anti-cancer properties. It is common for women to have elevated levels of estradiol and decreased levels of estriol. Supplementing estriol only with progesterone is a safer approach many times instead of supplementing estradiol and estriol levels.

Both estriol and estradiol can be used in bio-identical formulations. I recommend four times more estriol than estradiol in menopausal women as estriol will occupy the estrogen receptor sites and keeps the more potentially carcinogenic estrone and estradiol from causing a problem at the receptor site. Estrone and estradiol share a common pool together and, depending on the needs of an individual, can enzymatically change from one to the other. This pool helps balance the amount of estrogen available for an individual. To get rid of excess estrogen and for detoxification, estrogen goes through a process called *hydroxylation.* Hydroxylation (adding and OH-group) makes the hormone more water-soluble so that it can be eliminated through the sweat, urine, or stool. In the case of estrone, this hydroxylation process forms three metabolites: 2-hydroxyestrone, 16-alpha-hydroxyestrone, or 4-hydroxyestrone. If a person has a normal metabolism, fifty percent is converted to 2-hydroxyestrone (benign), forty percent is converted to 16-alpha-hydroxyestrone (carcinogenic), and ten percent is converted to 4-hydroxyestrone (carcinogenic). However, this ratio can change due to genetic variances in which increased percentages of either 16-alpha-hydroxyestrone or 4-hydroxyestrone occur, increasing breast cancer risk.

Phase I Estrogen Detoxification - Hydroxylation (-OH)

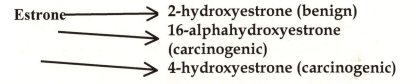

Estrone ⟶ **2-hydroxyestrone (benign)**
⟶ **16-alphahydroxyestrone (carcinogenic)**
⟶ **4-hydroxyestrone (carcinogenic)**

The second phase of estrogen detoxification is called *methylation.* This occurs when a methyl group (CH + 3) is added to the metabolites making them benign. When the methyl group is added to the hydroxyl group, the metabolite becomes benign. Genes play an important role in estrogen detoxification and explains why, if the body can produce a benign metabolite, such as 2-hydroxyestrone, it produces carcinogenic forms, such as 16-alpha-hydroxyestrone and 4-hydroxyestrone. Gene variation explains this. When the 2-, 4-, and 16-alpha-hydroxyestrone metabolites are out of balance and fail to methylate, there is increased risk for either breast cancer or osteoporosis: 2-hydroestrone is a weaker binding estrogen compared to 16-alpha-hydroxyestrone. This is why it is important to have more 2-hydroxyestrone than 16-alpha-hydroxyestrone. Higher levels of 2-hydroxyestrone relative to 16-alpha-hydroxyestrone decrease the risk for breast cancer.

Phase II: -Methylation (CH3+)

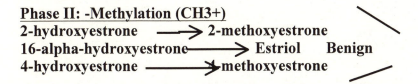

2-hydroxyestrone ⟶ 2-methoxyestrone
16-alpha-hydroxyestrone ⟶ Estriol   Benign
4-hydroxyestrone ⟶ methoxyestrone

However, levels of 2-hydroxyestrone that are too high relative to 16-alpha-hydroxyestrone can increase osteoporosis risk. Like many things in nature, balance is necessary. The rate of 2:16 is also important in the survivability and risk for breast cancer recurrence. The survival for women with breast cancer is only half for those with a ration of 2:16 of less than one compared to those with normal ratios. A normal ratio consist of as much of 2-hydroxyestrone as there are 16-alpha-hydroxyestrone, or slightly more, a 1:1 ratio, or a 1+:1 ratio, is better. When the 2-hydroxyestrone ratio is less than one, there is a thirty percent increased risk for breast cancer. It is easier to raise 2-hydroxyestrone levels than to lower 16-alpha-hydroxyestrone levels. We raise the 2-hydroxyestrone with supplements of flaxseed, omega 3 fatty acids, soy isoflavones, rosemary, turmeric, kudzu, strenuous exercise, weight loss, *chrysin* (a naturally occurring flavonoid), *indole-3-carbinol* (I-3-C) (compound found in cabbage, broccoli, Brussels sprouts, cauliflower, and kale), and *diindolylmethane* (DIM) (derived from I-3-C). Research has shown that supplementing 400 mg of I-3-C can cause an increase in the 2:16 ratio by as much as sixty-six percent.

Some polymorphism gene variants make estrogen detoxification impossible. Other polymorphisms can make the second phase, methylation, more difficult. These polymorphisms cause a buildup of toxic intermediate metabolites that have a negative impact on health and longevity. Specific nutrients—such as folic acid, B6, and B12—make a tremendous difference in these genetic predispositions.

In a normal metabolism, fifty percent of the time the hydroxyl group is placed in the 2 position, forty percent of the time in the 16 position, and ten percent of the time in the 4 position. Genetic variance increases the predisposition of placement into either the 16 or 4 position. For example, twenty eight percent of the population has a genetic predisposition to place an increased rate of hydroxyl in the 4 position.

The most common form of polymorphism, or gene variant, is called a *SNP (Single Nucleotide Polymorphism)*. The good news is that eighty to ninety percent of SNP's are unimportant. The bad news is that ten to twenty percent of these are clinically significant. The changes always occur in the enzymes, rendering the metabolic process dysfunctional. These variants can have a tremendous impact on our ability to utilize folic acid, riboflavin, B12, antioxidants, CoQ10, I-3-C, and other supplements. Twenty percent of the population has a detoxification gene variant called *CYP1A1* (a member of the largest family of *CYP450* detoxification enzymes). This causes those who carry this gene variant to produce reduced amounts of 2-hydroxyestrone, have decreased ability to metabolize acetaminophen, and have decreased detoxification with sulforaphanes like broccoli and Brussels sprouts. Two percent of the population has a *CYP1B1* (another member of the CYP 450 enzyme family) gene variant that causes increased formation of 4-hydroxyestrone, which increases breast, ovarian, uterine, head, and neck cancers. However, many people who have this variant never express the negative epigenetics because they take in more of specific nutrients—such as folic acid, B6, B12, DIM, and glutathione—needed to down regulate the epigenetic expression.

Sex Hormone Pathway Enzymes

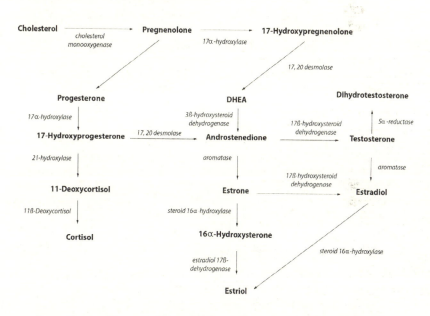

Genetic testing provides information about all these gene variants so that they can be addressed. This means that the individual can take specific positive actions to negate the expression. Smoking increases the expression of the CYP1B1 gene without adequate extra nutritional support. The gene variant increases the risk of breast cancer by thirteenfold. Cruciferous vegetables—such as broccoli, cauliflower, Brussels sprouts, and kale—and supplements like DIM and I-3-Carbonal promote the breakdown of estrone to the 2 position, improving the 2:16 ratio, and inhibit the expression of the CYP1A1 gene variant. Supplementation of resveratrol from red wine and DHEA inhibits the induced expression of the CYPIBI gene variant. Reducing the amount of body burden from the *xenoestrogens* from plastics and pesticides in the body is also important. The *COMT* (catechol-o-methyl transferase) polymorphism is critical as it reduces the effectiveness of the phase II estrogen detoxification, which is the methylation process. This is the process that turns the carcinogenic 4- and 16-alpha-hydroxyestrone metabolites into 16 and 4-methoxyestrone, which are not carcinogenic. You can review how these enzymes are involved in the estrogen detoxification process in the Estrogen Detoxification illustration.

The COMT polymorphism reduces the effectiveness of the phase I estrogen detoxification process by three to four hundred percent, which increases the risk for breast cancer if not compensated for by B Vitamin supplementation. This is why large amounts of folic acid, B6, and B12 supplementation are needed for these individuals. Estrogen detoxification pathways require B Vitamins. This is significant because it is estimated that eighty percent of Americans are deficient in one or more B Vitamins. An indirect way to measure the body's ability to methylate is by checking *homocysteine* (a non-protein alpha amino acid) levels. However, a better measure of methylation capacity by the body is through urinary *methylmalonic acid*. Treatments for the COMT polymorphism are increasing the consumption of cruciferous vegetables (broccoli, cauliflower, Brussels sprouts, and kale), garlic, onions, magnesium, *NAC,* Vitamin E, glutathione, *glutamine* and *glycine.*

GST, Glutathione-S-transferase is an important enzyme in phase II estrogen detoxification, acts as a powerful antioxidant, making the molecule more water soluble by adding sulfur. It

Estrogen Detoxification

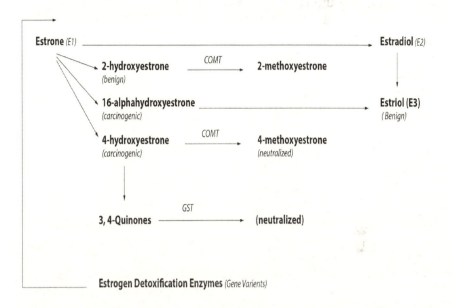

Estrone *(E1)* ── Estradiol *(E2)*

2-hydroxyestrone ──*COMT*──→ 2-methoxyestrone
(benign)

16-alphahydroxyestrone ·· Estriol **(E3)**
(carcinogenic)   *(Benign)*

4-hydroxyestrone ──*COMT*──→ 4-methoxyestrone
(carcinogenic)   *(neutralized)*

3, 4-Quinones ──*GST*········→ (neutralized)

Estrogen Detoxification Enzymes *(Gene Varients)*

making the molecule more water-soluble by adding sulfur. It metabolizes carcinogenic genomes. The gene variant involving GST is very significant effecting forty percent of European Americans, twenty-two percent of African-Americans, and fourteen percent of Asian Americans. Glutathione supplementation with sublingual liposome technology is necessary to negate the gene expression. This is an important gene variant to test for.

There are many polymorphisms involving estrogen detoxification. This is a commonly overlooked area by many doctors doing bio-identical hormone treatment. Appropriate supplementation is essential to deal with the many gene variants. Fortunately for us, the solutions have already been worked out.

The Case of Hot Flashes and Vaginal Dryness

This is a case study of two conditions that are the most common among peri-menopausal and post-menopausal women. The good news is that hot flashes and vaginal dryness respond very well to these protocols and without dangerous prescription medications.

D.L. was a fifty-five-year-old female physician who came to me complaining of twenty or more hot flashes per day and vaginal dryness. The hot flashes were adversely affecting her work with patients, and she reported her hot flashes were worse at night. These nightly hot flashes were accompanied with sweats that caused sleep interruptions multiple times throughout the night. She also complained of alternating periods of extreme cold. Alternating symptoms of hot and cold is often a sign of adrenal fatigue. Hot flashes are caused by periodic bursts of large amounts of estradiol, instead of the normal smooth sloping pattern of the hormone, which creates vasodilation of the blood vessels all over the body.

What most doctors don't tell their female patients is that hot flashes can last a long time. Depending upon how early they begin, hot flashes can last anywhere from 3.8 years to 11.57 years according to a study of 435 women in the Pennsylvania Ovarian Aging Study.[22] The study found that the younger a woman began experiencing hot flashes, the longer they lasted. If a woman began experiencing hot flashes before the age of forty to age forty-five, they lasted on an average of over 11 years. If they began between the ages of forty-five to fifty, the average length of time they continued was for 8.1 years. However, if the hot flashes began after the age of fifty, the average length of duration was 3.8 years. None of these sound like much fun to me.

A saliva hormone test and dried blood spot test for the thyroid were ordered. Thyroid levels were in the upper quintile (33%), and basal body temperature readings over five days averaged 97.8 degrees. These readings are considered acceptable. Salivary testing revealed extremely low progesterone, DHEA, cortisol, and estriol levels. Her estradiol and testosterone levels were acceptable, but estrone levels were slightly elevated. I recommended transdermal supplementation for pregnenolone (converts to progesterone and DHEA, both of which were low), DHEA, and progesterone. She also needed supplementation of sublingual B Vitamins to assure adequate estrogen methylation detoxification, DIM, I-3-C, and more to encourage the conversion of estrone to 2-hydroxyestrone (benign form), and a nutraceutical for adrenal support. In addition, she was given a high potency liquid extract of Pueraria Murifica, an herb from Thailand that converts easily to estriol.

Within two weeks, the patient reported her hot flashes, night sweats, and vaginal dryness were seventy-five percent improved. After about one month, the patient reported all symptoms were resolved. These results are typical for the symptoms of hot flashes and vaginal dryness in eighty to ninety percent of the women treated with similar protocols.

Case Study of Loss of Libido, Vaginal Dryness, Extreme Fatigue, and B12 Deficiency

L.P. was a fifty-nine-year-old post-menopausal female who, since age fifty-five, had complained of dry hair, skin, and vagina. She indicated that she had told her treating chiropractor that she was curious about bio-identical hormones, so her D.C. referred her to me for a consultation. She had a history of low B12 and also complained of chronic fatigue along with a loss of libido. Despite her fatigue, she indicated she did thirty minutes of treadmill cardiovascular exercise each week and lifted weights and did floor exercises. Bone density was reported to be normal. She had just had blood chemistries ordered by her medical doctor, which included a TSH. It was reported to her by her M.D. be within reference range. I asked her to check her basal body temperature readings for five mornings and ordered a saliva hormone test. She called in her basal body temperature results. Her average temperature was 96.3 F (normal is 98.6) first thing in the morning. She was hypothyroid, which meant that it was likely that most of her sex hormone levels were reduced.

The saliva hormone test confirmed low levels of progesterone, estradiol, estriol, DHEA, testosterone, and cortisol. There are always abnormal cortisol levels with low thyroid. With low cortisol levels, there is a reduction in DHEA. Her estrone levels were elevated, which increased her risk of having excess 16-apha-hydroxyestrone and/or 4-hydroxyestrone metabolites. You may recall that these are the carcinogenic metabolites while the 2-hydroxyestrone is the benign metabolite.

I recommended L.P. start transdermal pregnenolone, progesterone, DHEA, and estradiol/estriol in a 1:4 ratio, nutraceuticals for adrenal and thyroid support, sublingual liquid B Vitamins for methylation protection, and a nutraceutical containing DIM, I-3-C, chrysin, *peperine*, and more to encourage more 2-hydroxyestrone formation, increasing the 2:16 ratio. Increasing progesterone, estriol, B Vitamins, and the DIM/I-3-C reduce risk for estrogen related cancers of the breast, ovaries, and uterus. The support of the adrenal and thyroid along with the B Vitamins increases energy.

After two weeks, she was seen again for follow-up and reported her energy level was moderately improved, her skin and hair seemed less dry, and sex was much less painful. In the next two-week follow-up exam, she reported more improvement in all the same areas. She continued the same regimen for the next two months and was re-evaluated with saliva hormone testing. Progesterone, estradiol, estriol, DHEA levels were all more youthful. Cortisol was improved. She was advised that it often takes one to two years for the adrenals and/or thyroid gland to fully return to optimal function. However, in just a few weeks she was feeling more energetic and her libido had returned.

Take the estrogen self-assessment test to help determine if your estrogen levels are imbalanced.

ESTROGEN SELF-ASSESSMENT [1]
(Used with permission of author)

Estrogen Deficiency Symptoms
If supplementation has begun, increase dosage.

Sagging breasts
Lack of libido
Vaginal dryness
Urinary incontinence, infection
Hot flashes
Night sweats
Memory problems
Fuzzy thinking
Irregular menstrual cycles
Lack of menstruation
More wrinkles and skin aging
Increased insulin resistance

Estrogen Excess Symptoms
If supplementation has begun, decrease dosage.

Water retention
Cervical dysplasia, fibroids
Cancer
Hypothyroidism
Fatigue
Poor sleep
Bloating
Anxiety, fear
Breasts-swollen, tender
Severe headaches
Excess menstrual bleeding
Weight loss

Chapter12 References

1. Tai PL. *8 Powerful Secrets to Anti-Aging*. Dearborn, MI: Health Secrets; 2007.
2. Pgu U, Bradlow HL, Lvitz M. Estriol-3-sulfate in human breast cyst fluid concentration, possible pregnancy and physiological implications. *Ann NY Acad Sci* 1990: 586.83-7
3. Canani C, Qin K, Simoni M, et al. Testosterone and estradiol in a men with aromatase deficiency. *New England Journal of Medicine* 1997 Jul 10; 33: 91-95.
4. Behl C, Wickman M, Trapp T, Hodesboer R. 17-Beta estradiol protects neurons from oxidative stress induced cell death in vitro. *Biochem Biophys Res Commun,* 1995 Nov; 216 (2):473-82.
5. Docema SI, Husband C, O'Donnell ME, Barwin RN, Woodend AK. Estrogen related mood disorders reproductive life cycle factors. *Ans Ad Nur Sci* 2005; 28 (4) 3:364-5.
6. Lasuik GC, Hegidiren KM. The effects of estradiol on the central serotonergic system and its relationship to mood in women. *Biol Res Nurs* 2007 Oct; 9(2):167-60.
7. Head, K. Estriol, safety and efficacy. *Altern Med Rev* 1998; 3(2):01-3
8. Yang TS, Tsan SH, Chang SP, NG HT. Efficacy and safety of estriol replacement therapy for climacteric women. *Zhonghua Yi Xue Za Zhi (Taipei),* 1995 May; 55 (5): 386-91.
9. Tzinjouris VA, Aksu MF, Greenblait RB. Estriol, in the management of menopause. *JAMA* 1978 Apr 21; 239 (16): 1638-1641.
10. Raz, R, Stamm, WE. A controlled trial of intravaginal estriol in postmenopausal women with urinary tract infections. *NEJM* 1993 Sep 9; 329 (1): 753-56.
11. Collins, J. *What is Your Menopause Type?* Roseville, CA: Prima Health; 2000.
12. van der Linden MC, Gerretsen G, Brandhorst MS, Ooms EC, Kramer CM, Doesburg WH. The effect of estriol on the etiology of urethra symptoms. *EUNJ. Obstet Gynecol Reproduced Bio* 1993; 51(1): 29:33.

13. Sharpe RM. The role of estrogen in the male. *TEM* 1998 Nov 9; (9): 371-7.

14. Schober JM, Pfoff D. The Neurophysiology of Sexual Arousal. *Best Practice & Research Clinical Endocrinology & Metabolism* 2007 Sept: 21(3): 445-61.

15. Jankowska EA, Rozentryt P, Ponikowska B, et al. Circulating estradiol and mortality in men with systolic chronic heart failure. *JAMA* 2009 May 13; 301(18);1892-901.

16. Rochira V, Zirilli L, Maffei L, et al. Tall stature without growth hormone: four male patients with aromatase deficiency. *J Endocrinol Metab* 2010 Apr; 95(4): 1626-33.

17. Sherman AM, Cupples A, Demussie S, et al. Association of Estrogen Receptor Alpha Gene Variation and Cardiovascular Disease. *JAMA* 2003; 290(17): 2263-2270.

18. Hormones, Anthropometric Parameters, and Age in Hypogonadal Men Treated 1Year with a Perneatin-Enhanced Testosterone Transdermal System. *Journal of Clinical Endocrinology & Metabolism* 2000, May 12.

19. Schneider G, Kirshner MA, Berkowitz R, et al. Increased Estrogen Production in Obese Men. *Journal of Clinical Endocrinology & Metabolism* 1979 Apr; 48(4); 633-8.

20. Elias SA, Valenta LJ, Domurat ES. Male hypogonadism due to non-tumorous hyperestrogenism. *J Androl* 1990-N.

21. Fitzpatrick LA, Turner RT, Ritman ER, et al. Endochondral bone formation in the heart: a possible mechanism of coronary calcification. *Endocrinology* 2003 Jun; 144(6): 2214-9.

22. Freeman EW, Sammel MD. Methods in a longitudinal cohort study of late reproductive age women: the Penn Ovarian Aging Study (POAS). *Women's Mid-Life Health* 2016; 2:1 *DOI 10.1186/s40695-016-0014-2.*

23. Williams RJ, Biochemical individuality: the basis for the genetrophic concept. Oxford, England. (PysINFO Database Record © 2012 APA).

24. Prasher B, Negi S, Aggrwal S, et al. Whole genome expression and biochemical correlation of extreme constitutional types defied by Ayurveda. *Journal of Translational Medicine* 2008; 6:48.

25. Hon J, Zhang W, Cao H, Chen S, Wang Y. Genetic diversity and biography of the traditional Chinese Medicine, Gardenia jasminoides, based on ALF markers. *Biochemical Systematics and Ecology* 2007 Mar 3; 35(3); 138-145.

26. Galton DJ. Greek theories on eugenics. *J. Med Ethics* 1998; 24: 263-267.

27. Martucci CP, Fishman J. P450 enzymes of estrogen metabolism. *Pharmacology & Therapeutics* 1993; 57(2-3); 237-257.

28. Zimarina TS, Kristensen VN, Imyanitov EN, Berstein LM. Polymorphisms of *CYP1B1* and *COMT* in Breast and Endometrial Cancer. *Molecular Biology* 2004 May; 38(3):322-328.

29. Huang Cs, Chen HD, Chang KJ, Cheng CW, Hsu Sm, Shen CY. Breast Cancer Risk Associated with Genotype Polymorphism of the Estrogen-metabolizing Genes *CYP17, CYP1A1*, and COMT: A Multigenic Sudy on Cancer Susceptibility. *Cancer Res* 1999 Oct 1 59; 4870.

30. Hall DC. *Nutritional Influences on Estrogen Metabolism: A Summary*. Advanced Nutrition Publications © 2002.

31. Brignall M. Prevention and treatment of cancer with indole-3-carbinol. *Alternative Medicine Review* Dec 2001; 580+ AcademicOneFile. Web 17 May 2016.

32. Hashibe M, Brennan P, Strange R, et al. Meta- and Pooled Analyses of *GSTM1, GSTT1, GSTP1*, and *Cyp1A1* Genotype and Risk of Head and Neck Cancer. *Cancer Epidemiol Biomarkers Prev* 2003 Dec 1; 12:1509.

33. Ping J, Wang H, Huang M, Liu ZS. Genetic Analysis of Glutathione S-transferase A1 Polymorphism in the Chinese Population and the Influence of Genotype on Enzymatic Properties. *Toxicol Sci* 2006 Feb; 89(2): 438-443. *Doi: 10.1093/toxsci/kfj037.*

34. Lin HJ, Han CY, Bernstein DA, et al. Ethnic distribution of the glutathione-s-transferase Mu1-1 (GSTM1) null genotype in 1473 individuals and application to bladder susceptibility. *Carcinogenesis* 1994; 15(5): 1077-1081. *Doi: 10.1093/carcin/15.5.1077.*

13: Growth Hormone

Growth hormone (GH) is also known as *somatotropin*. It is produced by the anterior pituitary, but is controlled by the hypothalamus, the monitor of all internal sensory data in the body. Growth hormone levels are regulated by the hypothalamus through the release of two opposite functioning hormones. Growth hormone release-inhibiting hormone stimulates GH release, and somatotropin release-inhibiting hormone inhibits GH release.

Growth hormone is known as the *battery hormone*.[1] Growth hormone works both directly and indirectly on every cell in the body as it is a *master hormone*. GH binds directly to specific receptors in muscle, connective tissue (tendons, ligaments, bone, and fat) as well as every organ.[2] Growth factor is broken down by the liver, which then produces six human growth factors known as Insulin Growth Factor-1 (*IGF-1*), Insulin Growth Factor II (*IGF-2*), Epidermal Growth Factor (*EGF*), Vascular Growth Factor (*VGF*), Neural Growth Factor (*NGF*), and Transfer Growth Factor (*TGF*). Because there are also receptors throughout the body for these growth factors, these are considered an indirect influence of GH. IGF-1 is the best studied of all the growth factors. The thyroid hormones are essential in the production of IGF-1. Growth hormone secretion occurs in the early hours of the morning in a pulsatile method following a circadian (daily) rhythm. GH has an extremely short *half-life* of only minutes. Because GH is usually secreted about 3:00 AM and is only around for such a short duration, lab tests for evaluating it are not practical. However, IGF-1 has a half-life of about eighteen to twenty hours, so it can be readily monitored through laboratory tests. Research has demonstrated that GH and IGF-1 levels parallel each other.[1]

GH peaks during a person's growth spurt, reaching levels of 600-800 ng/ml or more. The level of GH secretion declines by fifty percent every seven years after eighteen to twenty-five years of age.[3] A fifty percent decrease in the secretion of GH/IGF 1 is commonly called *somatopause*. This decrease correlates with several negative symptoms that are associated with the aging process. Reduced GH/IGF-1 levels have been shown to cause sleeping pattern disorders, bone fragility, and central obesity (fat deposits around the abdomen and middle of the body). The decrease in GH/IGF-1 results in a decrease in muscle size, strength, and endurance, and cognition.[2-11]Normal levels of IGF-1 in an adult over age thirty range from 200-500 ng/ml. Only five percent of men and women under the age of forty have levels as low as 250 ng/ml. On average, by age fifty, half of the growth factor levels are depleted.[1] By age eighty, almost all are gone.[1] One third of individuals over age of fifty years of age show abnormal levels less than 200 ng/ml.[1] Like all other hormones, there is a big difference in physiological function having GH levels at 500 ng/ml vs. 200 ng/ml even though both levels are in the reference range.

When I had my IGF-1 tested at age fifty-two, I was low— below 200 ng/ml. This was despite the fact that I was under fifteen percent body fat, lifted weights four times/week, and ran three times/week. I elected to do GH injections. I started supplementing GH after I received stem cells for a left rotator cuff tear and right knee cartilage tear. I continued GH injections for approximately eighteen months. I generally felt more youthful in all aspects: physical strength and endurance, cognitive function, and libido. My skin was thicker and plumper. It improved my male pattern baldness to a certain extent. It seemed to reverse some of the grey in my hair. However, I seemed to have some edema in my face and hands and mild symptoms of carpal tunnel syndrome. These are fairly common symptoms, remedied by decreasing the dosage of GH.

In 1990, a landmark study by Pudman and colleagues provided the first evidence that GH supplementation in elderly could reduce and reverse some of the symptoms associated with somatopause.[2,27] Despite this study and others, exogenous GH therapy has been both controversial,[2-12]and costly.[28-31]Overall, in my case, the benefits far outweighed the negatives. The cost of the HG injection was approximately $500/month. It was money well-spent as far I am concerned.

There are additional documented positive benefits from supplementing HGH: Taking GH generally improves cholesterol levels, vision, immune system function, balance, thickening of skin, disease resistance, wound healing, organ function in the heart, kidney, liver, and sense of well-being.[1] In addition, greater cardiac output, amplified muscle mass, enhanced memory, enhanced libido, better sleep, increased burning of fat, increased muscle and bone strength, regrowth of hair, lowering of blood pressure, and improvement of social skills have been noted.

I no longer take GH injections as I have been able to effectively improve function without the injections. There are several effective ways of naturally stimulated HG/IF-1 levels and function by eliminating or decreasing a number of lifestyle factors that have been found to decrease GH and IGF-1 secretion. There are multiple studies to demonstrate that trunk obesity accurately predicts decreased GH levels.[2] Also, there are numerous studies showing that poor nutritional status, sleep reduction, and deconditioning from lack of exercise all affect GH and IGF-1 levels regardless of age.[2] Individually, or in combination, each of these factors negatively affect muscle/fat ratios, bone strength, endurance, and cognitive function, independent of their effects on GH/IGF-1 levels. It is evident that an unhealthy lifestyle contributes to somatopause, just as it contributes to menopause and *andropause* (the male version of menopause). These negative lifestyle habits cause profound reduction in the GH/IGF-1 secretion as well as indirectly by the promotion of an accelerated physical aging and psychological symptoms.

Healthy lifestyles changes have been shown to increase endogenous GH/IGF-1 production through a variety of ways. Some of the most important methods for increasing GH/IGF-1 levels include decreasing central obesity, avoiding meals with a high glycemic load, getting adequate sleep, doing high intensity exercise, and having a higher protein, lower glycemic meal for your last meal of the day.[2] Fortunately, it has been shown by research that GH/IGF-1 secretion can be partially reversed with weight loss.[8] However, trunk and visceral fat are often an indicator of both insulin and leptin resistance and often need to be corrected for weight loss to occur. High glycemic meals consisting of white bread, sugary cereals, white rice, white potatoes, potato chips, cookies, sodas, and fruit juices cause increased insulin production that is a direct inhibitor of GH/IGF-1 secretion. Research illustrates that inadequate sleep, irregular sleeping patterns, and poor quality sleep can reduce GH secretion substantially.[3,6] To optimize sleep, keep a regular bedtime (preferably by 10 PM) and wake up time, allowing seven or more hours, do not consume caffeine four to six hours before bedtime, do not consume more than one alcoholic beverage before bedtime, and keep excess noise and light out of the bedroom.

Exercising at eighty percent of your maximum heart rate will help your reach lactic acid threshold, causing subsequent GH release. Several studies have shown that circuit training, which utilizes relatively light resistances, can be just as effective at driving GH secretion as more intense powerlifting. Circuit training usually entails increased number of repetitions per set (fifteen to twenty), and rest periods are usually under thirty seconds. If you like longer duration low intensity "cardio" training like jogging, cycling, or swimming, you need to supplement with short bursts or sprints every four to five minutes to maximize GH release. Exercising above the lactate threshold of eighty percent of the maximum heart rate (220 - number of years old you are x .80) appears to increase total secretion of GH for at least twenty-four hours.

There have seen a number of oral nutrients that have shown promise in raising serum GH levels. One of these is a compound named GDP-choline, which has shown in one study that administration caused a dramatic fourfold increase in serum GH levels compared to baseline levels. The most abundant amino acid (protein building block) in the body is glutamine. Oral doses of 2000 mg have been shown to increase plasma GH levels.[2,7] Oral intake of arginine also increases the release of GH. When arginine is combined with exercise even greater amounts of GH are measured. Ornithine and alpha-ketoglutarate have been reported to increase GH secretion as well. The amino acid, glycine, has been shown to improve the quality of sleep and increase GH secretion when taken before bedtime.

To summarize, safe methods for enhancing endogenous GH production include the following:

- losing excess abdominal fat,
- avoiding high glycemic meals,
- good sleep habits,
- eating a higher protein, lower carbohydrate meal at bedtime, and
- exercising regularly to your lactate acid threshold, which is usually about 80% of your maximum heart rate.

In addition, specific nutrients, including GDP-choline, arginine, ornithine, glycine, glutamine, and niacin (B3) can help increase your endogenous GH secretion. Fortunately for you, there is an even easier way to naturally boost your GH/IGF levels than the use of the *secretagogues* (herbs or nutrients that facilitate hormone production) mentioned above. There is a technological breakthrough of using a water extraction of deer velvet antler, a natural source of not only IGF-1, but also the other five growth factors, IGF-2, EGF, VGF, NGF, and TGF, I wrote about earlier in the chapter. This process has been enhanced by a sublingual delivery system using liposome technology. Using this *nanotechnology*, you get the benefits of the human hormone growth factor without the inconvenience of HGH injection and at a fraction of the cost (about fifteen percent of what I was paying for GH injections). Take this growth hormone self-assessment test to help determine if you are suffering from an excess or deficiency.

HGH ASSESSMENT [1]
(Used by permission of author)

HGH Deficiency
If supplementation has already been taken, increase dosage.

Waist and hip fat
Loss of strength
Loss of muscle
Increase fatigue
Bone, joint pain
No sexual interest
Anti-social behavior
Thinning, sagging, wrinkling skin
Lack of libido

HGH Excess
If supplementation has already been taken, decrease dosage.

Carpal tunnel syndrome
Sudden arthritis pain
Water retention
High blood pressure
Prostate pain, enlargement
Aggressive behavior

Chapter 13 References

1. Tai PL. *8 Powerful Secrets to Anti-Aging*. Dearborn Heights, MI: Health Secrets USA; 2007.
2. Enhancing Growth Hormone Naturally. *Life Extension Magazine*, 2009, Mar.
3. Gentili A, Adler RA. Growth Hormone Replacement in Older Men Differential Diagnosis. *Medscape News & Perspective.* http:/emedicine.medscape.com/article/126999-oneness.
4. de Boer H, Blok GJ, van der Veen EA. Clinical aspects of growth hormone aging and growth hormone status deficiency in adults. *Endocr. Rev.* 1995 Feb; 16(1): 63-86.
5. Santorio A, Conti A, Molinare E, et al. Growth, growth hormone and cognitive functions. *Horm Res*1996; 45 (1-2): 23-9.
6. Toogood AA, Shalet SM. Aging and growth hormone status. *Baillieres Clin Endocrinol Metab*1998 Jul; 12(2): 281-96.
7. Van Cauter E, Leproult R, Plat L, Age related changes in slow wave sleep and REM Sleep and relationship with growth hormone and cortisol levels in healthy men. *JAMA,* 2000 Aug 16; 284(7):861-8.
8. Alemar A, de Vries WR, de Haan EH, et al. Age sensitive cognitive function,growth hormone and insulin like growth factor/plasma levels in healthy older men. *Neuropsychobiology* 2000 Jan; 41(2):73-8.
9. Compton DM, Bachman LD, Brand D, Aket TL. Age associated changes in cognitive function in highly educated adults: emerging myths and realities. *Int. J Geriatr Psychiatry,* 2000 Jan 15(1): 75-78.
10. Van Dam PS, Aleman, A, de Vries WR, et al. Growth hormone, insulin-like growth factor, and cognitive function in adults. *Growth Horm IGF Res* 2000 Apr; 10: (Suppl.B): 569-573.
11. Scheider HJ, Pagotto LL, Stalla GK. Central effects of the somatotropic system. *Eur J Endocrinol* 2003 Nov. 149 (5): 377-92.

12. Scheider HJ, Pagotto LL, Stalla GK. Central effects of the somatotropic system. *Eur J Endocrinol* 2003 Nov 149 (5): 377-92.
13. Rudman D, Feller AG, Nagrai HS, et al. Effects of human growth hormone in men over 60 years old. *N Eng l J Med,* 1990 July 5: 323 (1): 1-6.
14. Sherlock M, Toogood AA, Aging and growth hormone/insulin like growth factor-1 axis. *Pituitary* 2007:10(2): 189-203.
15. Liu H, Bravata DM, Olkin I, et al. Systematic review: the safety and efficacy of growth hormone in the healthy elderly. *Annals Intern Med* 2007 Jan 16; 146(2): 104-15.
16. Giordano R, Bonelli L, Marinazzo E, Ghigo E, Arvat. Growth hormone treatment in human aging: benefits and risk. *Hormones (Athens)*, 2008 Apr: 7(2): 133-9.
17. Friedlander AL, Butterfield GE, Moynihan S, et al. One year of insulin-like growth factor 1 treatment does not affect bone density, body composition, or psychological measures in postmenopausal women. *J Clin Endocrinol Metab* 2001 Apr; 86(4) : 196-503.
18. Cummings DE, Merriam GR. Growth hormone therapy in adult. *Ann Rev Med* 2003; 54:513-33.
19. Clemmons DR. The relative roles of growth and IGF-1 in controlling insulin sensitivity. *J Clin Invest* 2003 Jan; 113 (1): 25-22.
20. Yuan K, Wareham N, Frystyk J, et al. Short term low dose growth hormone and menstruation in subjects with impaired glucose tolerance and the metabolic syndrome:effects on beta cell function and post load glucose tolerance. *Eur J Endocrinol* 2004 Jul; 15 1(1): 39-45.
21. Chan JM, Stampfer MJ, Giovannici E, et al. Plasma insulin-like growth factor-I and prostate cancer risk: a prospective study. *Science,* 1998 Jan 23; 279(5350): 563-6.
22. Shin M, Cohen P. IGFs and human cancer: Implications regarding the risk of growth hormone therapy. *Horm Res* 1999:5 1 (Suppl.3): 45-51.
23. Cohen P, Clemmons DR, Rosenfeld RG. Does the GH/IGF axis play a role in cancer pathogenesis? *Growth Horm IGF Res* 2000 Dec; 10(6): 297-305.

24. Khandwala HM, McCutcheon I., Flyvberg A, Friend KE. The effects of insulin like growth factors on tumorigenesis and neoplastic growth. *Endocrinol Rev* 2000 Jun; 2(3): 215-46.

25. Laban C, Bustin SA, Jenkins PJ, The GH-IGF 1 axis and breast cancer. *Trends Endocrinol Meta,* 2003 Jan: 14 (1): 28-34.

26. Ceda GP, Ceresini G, Denti, L, et al. Effects of cytidine 5'-diphosphocholine line administration on basal and growth hormone-releasing-induced hormone secretion in elderly patients. *Acta Endocrinol (Copenh)* 1991 May; 124 (5) : 516-20.

27. Rudman D, Feller AG, Hoskote S, et al. Effects Of Human Growth Hormone In Men Over 60 Years Old. *NEJM* 1990 Jul 5;323(1);1-6.

28. Welbourne TC. Increased plasma bicarbonate are growth hormone after oral glutamine load. *Am J Clin Nutr* 1995 May; 6. (5): 1068-61.

29. Cynober L. Ornithine alpha-ketoglutarate are potent processor of arginine and nitric oxide a new job for an old friend. *J Nutr* 2004.Oct; 136 (10 Suppl) 128588-28625 discussion 28955.

30. Chase MH. Confirmation of the glycinergic postsynaptic inhibition is responsible for the atonia of REM Sleep. *Sleep* 2008. Nov 1; 3 (11) 1487-90.

31. Ngondi JL, Matsinkou P, Oben JE. The use of Irvingia gabonesin extract (1G0B131) in the management of metabolic syndrome in Cameroon. 2008. Submitted for publication.

Chapter 14: Adrenals

The two adrenal glands are located superior and anterior to the two kidneys and look somewhat like a hat sitting on top of each kidney. The adrenal glands are composed of two different areas, the medulla and the cortex. There are three major classes of hormones produced in each of the three different zones of the adrenal cortex: mineralocorticoids, glucocorticoids, and the sex hormones. The outer most layer of the adrenal cortex is called the *zona glomerulosa* and produces aldosterone. The middle layer is called the *zona fasciculate* and produces cortisol. The innermost layer is the *zona reticularis,* where DHEA and androstenedione are manufactured.

The medulla, or the inner portion, is responsible for the production of the *catecholamines*, *epinephrine* and *norepinephrine*. Epinephrine is better known as adrenaline. These two chemicals, epinephrine and norepinephrine, are part of the autonomic (automatic) nervous system and are produced in response to stress. They are part of the fight or flight response.

Roughly eighty percent of the output from the adrenals is epinephrine (adrenaline) and the other twenty percent, norepinephrine. You produce these when you need more energy for emergencies, to think faster, to see better, and to cope with fears and anxieties. In today's world this mechanism is so overused that most forty-year-old Americans are already suffering from adrenal fatigue.

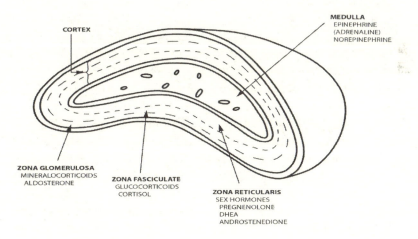

CORTEX

MEDULLA
EPINEPHRINE
(ADRENALINE)
NOREPINEPHRINE

ZONA GLOMERULOSA
MINERALOCORTICOIDS
ALDOSTERONE

ZONA FASCICULATE
GLUCOCORTICOIDS
CORTISOL

ZONA RETICULARIS
SEX HORMONES
PREGNENOLONE
DHEA
ANDROSTENEDIONE

Adrenal Gland

The adrenal gland is regulated directly by the pituitary that secretes ACTH (adrenocorticotropic hormone) that signals the adrenal cortex to produce and secrete cortisol. The pituitary is under the command of the hypothalamus, which secretes a releasing hormone to communicate to the pituitary. (See the Hypothalamus-Pituitary-Adrenal Axis chart in Chapter 7.) It is the job of the hypothalamus to monitor all internal sensory data, which includes blood hormone levels. If levels of cortisol are too low in the blood, the hypothalamus senses this and secretes more releasing hormone, which signals the pituitary to secrete more ACTH, which signals more cortisol production and secretion from the adrenal glands. Conversely, once cortisol levels are sufficient to handle the situation, the hypothalamus stops the secretion of releasing hormone, which causes cortisol production and secretion to cease. This is called a negative feedback system and is discussed in Chapter 2 in the first paragraph. It is very much like the thermostat in our homes that regulates the air temperature.

ACTH, secreted from the pituitary, stimulates cortisol production from the adrenal cortex. Cortisol is an anti-inflammatory. Eating causes your cortisol levels to elevate slightly. When you exercise, your cortisol levels elevate slightly to compensate for the inflammation created by the exercise. Cortisol levels in the saliva can be monitored to make sure you are not overtraining. If cortisol levels fail to rise after a significant workout, you must rest for a few days. Not resting may make you to go into adrenal fatigue, which will take weeks to months to recover. Cortisol can also create or remove bone mass from your body. With chronic cortisol production, you create excess glucose (sugar). If this excess glucose is not spent by significant physical activity, it is deposited as fat around your waist, middle, and visceral organs.

ACTH also plays a small part in the production of the mineralocorticoids like aldosterone. Aldosterone controls the fluid volume in the body. Aldosterone is responsible for the pressure and volume in our blood vessels, creating the *blood pressure.* Without ACTH to stimulate cortisol and aldosterone, your brain would not have adequate sugar or blood volume for optimum function when you stand. Improperly functioning ACTH signals or adrenal fatigue creates *postural hypotension.* This means that blood pressure is lower, instead of higher, in the standing position vs. the sitting or lying position. This abnormal finding is indicative of a H-P-A

(Hypothalamus-Pituitary-Adrenal) axis dysfunction. The symptoms of these are *light headedness*, dizziness, or disorientation for a few seconds, or longer, immediately upon standing from a sitting or lying position. This is fairly common in the elderly.

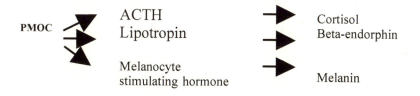

The *precursor* to ACTH is a protein named *proopiomelanocortin* (PMOC). Besides ACTH formation from PMOC, other fragments of the PMOC become lipotropin, which is a precursor for the beta-endorphins produced in the brain. These *opioid* peptides relieve pain and produce euphoric feelings. Melanocyte-stimulating hormone that controls the melanin pigmentation of the skin is also derived from the PMOC. See graph above.

In addition to the glucocorticoids (cortisol) and the mineralocorticoids (aldosterone), the sex hormones are also produced in the adrenal cortex. The gonads produce many of the sex hormones, but the adrenals do as well, particularly as we age. The production of a female's testosterone occurs in the cortex of the adrenals.

Adrenal fatigue is always found in all chronic illness. It is essential that the adrenal glands, as well as the thyroid, are working properly to allow the sex hormones to function properly. Epinephrine (adrenaline) and cortisol allow the cells in the body to work. Thyroid hormone determines the rate of cellular activity. It is the thyroid hormone that determines the size and number of mitochondria in the cell. The synthesis of epinephrine (adrenaline) and norepinephrine, as well as thyroid hormone, is dependent upon an amino acid, *tyrosine*. This conversion of tyrosine to epinephrine and norepinephrine takes place within the adrenal medulla. The adrenal glands and the thyroid function are very dependent upon Vitamin C and B Vitamins. It is interesting to note that the amino acid tyrosine is part of the whole vitamin C complex.

Adrenal fatigue is marked by a host of symptoms:

- alternating feelings of hot and cold,
- chronic fatigue,
- weakness,
- inability to deal with stress,
- immune problems,
- wake up in the middle of the night and unable to get back to sleep,
- anxiety,
- depression,
- chronic "itis" of some kind,
- blood sugar regulating problems,
- digestive problems,
- elevated cholesterol, and
- increased blood pressure.

The postural hypotension is a physical finding in patients with adrenal fatigue. This is called a positive *Ragland's test*, which is an abnormal finding of a lower blood pressure reading in the standing position vs. the lying position. Normally, the systolic number (upper number of blood pressure) should be six to ten points higher in the standing vs. lying position.

One of the best tests for monitoring adrenal function is with salivary testing of cortisol. I find very few patients over the age of forty with normal cortisol levels. The vast majority of middle-aged and elderly Americans have some level of adrenal fatigue. The extreme version of adrenal fatigue is known as *Addison's disease*. Addison's disease can be life threatening. Addison's disease is denoted by cardiovascular disease, lethargy, diarrhea, and weakness.

The opposite of Addison's disease is *Cushing's disease*, which is a chronic, prolonged production of cortisol denoted by moon face, osteoporosis, buffalo hump, diabetes, obesity, wrinkled skin, hypertension, a large abdominal area, and weakened muscles. Cushing's disease is the most prevalent disease involving cortisol. This condition is usually secondary to the destruction of the adrenal cortex by infection or autoimmune disease. Insufficient cortisol is often accompanied by aldosterone deficiency.

There are a number of nutrients and herbs that are important for adrenal support. Some of the key nutrients are Vitamin C, B Vitamins, especially pantothenic acid, tyrosine, and *adaptogens* such as *Astragalus* and *licorice root, protomorphogens* (usually bovine or sheep adrenal extracts without the hormones), and the *homeopathic, Adrenimium.* Consult a doctor who is familiar with both bio-identical therapy and nutrition for best results.

One of the key factors to correcting or preventing adrenal fatigue is sleep. The adrenal glands repair themselves between 10:00 PM and 4:00 AM. If you want your adrenal glands functioning optimally, you need sleep during this time. It has been my experience that the adrenal glands will not repair without adequate sleep. Try to be in bed by 10:00 PM. Most of us need seven to eight hours of quality sleep for good health. People who work the third shift are some of the sickest people in the world. Their hormone levels are low. They have more cancer. My advice to all my patients who work a night shift is to either switch to a daytime shift or find another job.

In summary, adrenal function is essential in having the endocrine (hormone) system working at its best. Many doctors who do hormone replacement therapy overlook adrenal function testing and the monitoring of cortisol levels.

Take the adrenal self-assessment test to help determine in your adrenal glands are functioning properly.

ADRENAL SELF-ASSESSMENT [1]
(Used with permission of author)

Cortisol Deficiency
If supplementation has already begun, increase dosage.

Insomnia
Fatigue
Digestive problem
Emotional imbalance
Loss of sexual interest
Low blood pressure

Cortisol Excess
If supplementation has already begun, decrease dosage.

Sleep problems
Sugar metabolism problems
Fat deposits
Osteoporosis
Lack of energy
Increased cholesterol, water retention

Slow heart beat
Feeling depressed
Light headedness when standing
from a lying or sitting position

Increased blood pressure
Thin skin
Loss of muscle mass

Anxiousness, irritability,
nervousness
Feeling of stress
Weight gain in trunk of body
Arthritis and muscle pain
Hair loss

Chapter 14 References

1. Tai PL. *8 Powerful Secrets to Anti-Aging.* Dearborn Heights, MI: Health Secrets; 2007.
2. Wilson JL. *Adrenal Fatigue: The 21st Century Stress Syndrome.* Petaluma, CA: Smart Publications; 2001.
3. Rosen, Joel. *Adrenal Fatigue Recovery.*
4. Tai PL. *Clinical Nutrition.* Dearborn Heights, MI: Health Secrets USA; pending publication.
5. Hansen F. *The Adrenal Fatigue Solution.* Perfect Health; 2016. http://adrenalfatiguesolution.com/get-started/. Accessed April 15, 2016.

The thyroid hormones are produced by a small butterfly-shaped organ located in the front of the throat area. The thyroid hormones are controlled by a negative feedback system involving the hypothalamus, pituitary, and the thyroid gland (H-P-T axis). See H-P-T axis chart below.

Hypothalamus-Pituitary-Thyroid (HPT) Axis

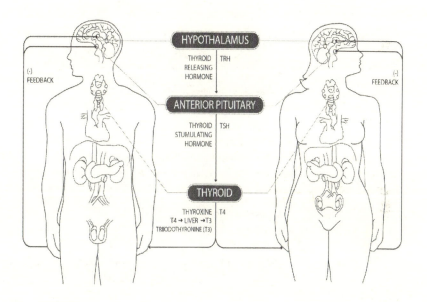

Thyroid hormones determine the rate, or how fast, the cells in the body work. Inherited function is passed on primarily by the mother. When the sperm fertilizes the egg, there are very few mitochondria contributed from the sperm. The vast majority of the mitochondria for this new fertilized ovum come from the mother's egg. The function of the thyroid determines the number and size of the mitochondria. Your mother's thyroid function affects your health potential. The mitochondria are where the ATP (*adenosine triphosphate*) energy is generated for each cell. Poor thyroid function equates to poor cellular energy and function.

By far, the most common abnormality of the thyroid gland is *hypothyroidism*. However, only about two percent of Americans have been clinically diagnosed. This number increases fivefold to ten percent when Americans over the age of sixty-five are assessed. This is another perfect example of the increasing number of hormone deficiencies as we age. Women are more susceptible to developing hypothyroidism than men. Some of the more common symptoms of low thyroid function include dry skin; dry, brittle, thinning hair; thinning of lateral third of the eyebrows; chronic constipation; sensitivity to cold; infertility; chronic fatigue; inability to lose weight despite a change in diet and exercise; and mental dullness and difficulty concentrating.

There are several experts in the area of thyroid like Dr. Broda Barnes and Dr. David Brownstein who feel there may be an alarming rate of as many as forty percent or more of the population who are undiagnosed with hypothyroidism. Based on my personal experience of over thirty-five years in practice with over fifteen thousand patients, I have to agree with Drs. Barnes and Brownstein. If forty percent of the U.S. population has an under-functioning thyroid, that is an epidemic.

Actually, hypothyroidism occurs worldwide. There is a western province in China where seventy-five percent of the population is hypothyroid and retarded as well. When China allowed The Special Olympics to come to their country a few years ago, they had over five hundred thousand participants throughout the country. Why would there be so many? There are negligible amounts of iodine in the soil and diet. Iodine is a key nutrient for the thyroid as well as the breast, uterus, ovaries and prostate, and it is critical in the brain development of a fetus. The uterus and breasts need as much iodine as the thyroid and this is one of the reasons why more women are hypothyroid than men. The iodine deficiency in the U.S., as well as many other minerals like zinc, is widening and worsening extending way beyond the *goiter belt* (the U.S. Midwest). U.S. government studies estimate that commercial farmlands have lost seventy-five percent of their mineral content. South America has a similar loss of minerals in the soil.

Other critical nutrients necessary for optimal thyroid function are selenium, zinc, B12, and Vitamin D. Nutritional deficiencies in one or more of these nutrients are common. In the past twenty-four months I have not evaluated one patient with a vitamin D level higher than 36 ng/ml (reference range is 30-100 ng/ml), and this is in Florida, "The Sunshine State".

Environmental factors also affect thyroid function negatively. Arsenic is often found in well water. Mercury, from amalgam fillings, large ocean fish, and high fructose corn syrup inhibit thyroid function. Another environmental factor that affects thyroid function is *BPA* (bisphenol A). BPA is found in many plastic products including bottled water, soda, and storage containers for leftovers. *Triclosan* is found in personal care products such as deodorant, toothpaste, mouthwash and shaving cream to reduce or prevent bacteria growth, and *4-nonylphenol* is found in detergent, carpet cleaners, pesticides, dry cleaning, cosmetics, paints and coatings, household products, and paper manufacturing.

Other chemicals can displace *iodine* in the body. Iodine is in the *halide* family in the elemental chemical chart. The other halides—*chlorine, bromine, and fluoride*—compete with iodine for the same receptor sites in the tissues of the body because of their similar molecular structure and *valence*. Chlorine is in our water supply. Bromine is in our new car interior, children and /or grandchildren's car seats, processed breads, some sports drinks, and Mountain Dew. There is fluoride in our toothpaste, mouthwash, and the water supply in some municipalities. Being deficient in iodine and being surrounded with chlorine, bromine, and fluoride is a bad combination. I have found toxic levels of bromine and fluoride in many of my patients through urinalysis. The analogy one of my mentors, Dr. Paul Tai, makes is that "Iodine is like a chimpanzee and chlorine, bromine, and fluoride are like gorillas. What chance does a chimpanzee have against a gorilla?" The more powerful chlorine, fluoride, and bromine molecules occupy many of the iodine receptor sites because of an iodine deficiency.

Through the years, I have consulted with hundreds of patients who had the classic symptoms of hypothyroidism. Most of these patients had their TSH (thyroid stimulating hormone produced by the pituitary) evaluated and had been assured by their doctor that their thyroid was perfectly normal. I had the patient check their basal body temperature first thing in the morning for five mornings. The normal temperature should be approximately 98.6 F first thing in the morning. All of these patients had subnormal temperatures. I treated the patient for low thyroid function with the appropriate nutrients, herbs and protomorphogens to support their thyroid and their adrenals. Almost everyone who has low thyroid function also has abnormal adrenal function as well. After taking the appropriate supplements, their health improved.

Thyroid function is critical for muscle function. The heart is the hardest working muscle in the body. Low thyroid function is a better predictor of heart attack than high cholesterol levels. In rating Cummulative Death's Hazard Rates in Cardiac Patients, the lower reference range T3 levels were a better predictor for cardiac death in patients than were elevated cholesterol and triglyceride levels. This is one reason why it is so important that the thyroid hormones be evaluated properly, especially when there are too many people that are undiagnosed with hypothyroidism.

Why wasn't the TSH in the blood showing the hypothyroidism? There are a number of possible explanations for this. The first problem is that a lab is only screening for TSH (thyroid stimulating hormone secreted by the pituitary) for thyroid function, and the reference range in most laboratories is much too broad. Many labs have a .45-4.5 mIU/L reference range, which equates to a one thousand percent difference between the low range of normal and the high range of normal. In addition, TSH levels can fluctuate as much as forty percent. Most doctors with a background in nutrition and/or functional medicine feel the TSH levels should be 1-2 mIU/L, at most 1-3 mIU/L, but certainly any value over 2 mIU/L is suspect in my mind and highly likely to indicate an under-functioning thyroid gland.

Another problem with only evaluating TSH is that it is a fragile hormone that breaks down quickly in serum. TSH should be measured immediately after the blood is drawn. If the blood was drawn at 8:00 am, and the test was not run until after lunch, much of the hormone could already have broken down. This would cause a false negative reading due to the breakdown of much of the TSH. In my opinion, it is necessary to evaluate the free T3 and free T4 levels, as well as reverse T3, *TRA*, and *TPO* levels to determine thyroid function.

What do T4 and T3 mean? T4 represents a molecular structure containing four iodine atoms, and T3 represents a molecular structure containing three iodine atoms. This cleaving of an iodine atom occurs in the liver requiring several nutrients like selenium, zinc, and B vitamins. If any of these key nutrients are missing, or the liver function is sub-par, there will be a lack of conversion into the bioactive form T3. T4 represents about ninety percent of the total circulating thyroid hormones. Elevated or high levels of T4 suggest that T4 is not converting to T3, the bioactive form. It is the T3 that activates the receptor site. T4 must be converted to T3 to bind to a receptor site.

Another potential problem can occur in the conversion process, often due to nutritional deficiencies, genetic variants, or environmental toxins. This conversion process causes one of the three iodine atoms to be placed on the inner ring vs. the outer ring of the T3 molecule. This particular aberration is known as *rT3* (reverse T3.) While it has the ability to occupy a thyroid receptor site, it cannot activate the appropriate cell activity. Therefore, the more rT3 produced, the more rT3 can bind to receptor sites, leaving no receptor available for the bio-active T3 form to bind to. If a doctor only orders a total T3 and not the free T3 and rT3, the overall reading may seem normal as there is no differentiation as to what kind of T3 it is. The total T3 includes the bound T3, free T3, and rT3.

The other readings that are important are called TPO (thyroid peroxidase) and TRA (thyroglobulin). TPO and TRA are auto-antibodies that attack the thyroid. The autoimmune diseases are also known as *thyroiditis* or Hashimoto's disease (hypo-function) or *Graves's* disease (hyper-function). These types of patients may not tolerate large doses of iodine initially. Supplementation of iodine must be slowly titrated and carefully monitored.

Another consideration in evaluating the potential hypothyroid patient is the realization that thyroid hormone levels are only fifty percent of the equation. The other fifty percent lies within the thyroid receptor in each cell. A patient with normal reference ranges of TSH, free T3, free T4, rT3, and TPO can still have functional hypothyroidism. This is due to thyroid receptor resistance, known as type II hypothyroidism. This type II hypothyroidism appears to be increasing in the population, most probably due to environmental toxicity factors. Thyroid resistance can be likened to insulin resistance, which you may have heard of. The thyroid receptor resistant individual will need rT3 levels to be reduced and free T3 levels to be optimum (upper quartile of the reference range) to effectively stimulate the receptor.

It has been my experience that I have never seen a hypothyroid patient who did not also have adrenal dysfunction as well. These patients always exhibit abnormal cortisol levels on saliva hormone testing. The adrenal glands must be treated concurrently with the thyroid to restore the endocrine (hormonal) balance. It is the cortisol that allows the cell to function, and the thyroid hormone that determines the speed with which the cell works. One hormone cannot function optimally without other.

Another important hormone produced by the thyroid gland is *calcitonin*. This hormone works with the parathyroid hormone to balance the calcium and phosphorous physiology. This homeostasis or maintenance of calcium in the blood occurs because of calcitonin's effects upon the bone, a great warehouse of calcium, and by its influence in the kidney regarding the control of how much calcium is lost or its ability to reabsorb calcium. Calcitonin also affects the small intestine in conjunction with Vitamin D to enhance the absorption of calcium contained in food. It also suppresses the resorption of bone by inhibition on the activity of *osteoclasts* (cells that take away old bone cells). Calcitonin's effects on the distal kidney tubules in the retention of calcium and phosphorous is similar to the effect aldosterone has on the distal tubules in the retention of sodium and potassium.

The most common medications prescribed by medical doctors for someone diagnosed with clinical hypothyroidism are *synthroid* or *Levothyroxine*. Both are synthetic forms of T4. Many patients who are placed on these medications do not feel any better after begin medicated, or feel better only temporarily. Often, the dose of the medication is increased over time. The reason for this is that the T4 is not converted into T3 because there is a deficiency of key elements like selenium, zinc, or B12, there is liver dysfunction, or the adrenal dysfunction has not been addressed.

A good option for many is Armor Thyroid, which is *dessicated* pig thyroid. This dessicated thyroid has T4 and T3 in an 80/20 ratio and also contains other necessary nutrients. It provides better physiological function for many. Most patients, however, respond to a combination of nutraceuticals, herbs, protomorphogens, and homeopathic formulas. A hypothyroid or a hypo-adrenal condition is not fixed overnight. It might easily take one or two years to repair a severely under-functioning thyroid or adrenal gland.

However, symptomatic changes can often be seen within two weeks.

Thyroid Case Study

One of the most dramatic cases of resolving a *goiter* I have ever seen was on my own sister. I had not seen her for approximately two months. My brother, sister, and I had met at that time to visit our mother in Ft. Smith, Arkansas. The next time I saw her was for our mother's funeral. As soon as I saw my sister, I asked her what was going on with her thyroid. It was huge! There was a goiter about the size of two to three prunes. It was quite apparent to me as I approached her from some fifteen to twenty feet away. She was unaware of it. It was probably present, though much smaller, two months prior, but I missed it. I recommended she get the dried blood spot test for thyroid done as soon as she got back to Albuquerque, New Mexico. In the meantime, I called the warehouse for some products to be shipped to her immediately. I sent her five different products—a blend of *cordyceps* mushrooms to help regulate her H-P-A axis and H-P-T axis and give liver support, a sublingual liquid B Vitamins complex, a supplement for adrenal support, some liquid iodine/iodide to help her body make T4, and a supplement that contained nutrients to help convert T4 to T3. The effect of this combination was dramatic and rapid. The goiter was shrunk seventy to eighty percent within thirty days and undetectable in sixty days. This demonstrates how critical specific micronutrients are to optimum endocrine function of organs like the thyroid.

The Case of the Man with Low Thyroid on Levothyroxine

This is a case of a fifty-two-year-old man who had been diagnosed with hypothyroidism five years prior and started on Levothyroxine, but never felt any significantly more energetic after taking the medications. B.M. had also been placed on Lipitor (a statin medication for elevated cholesterol) for ten years and Lisinopril (for hypertension) for seven years. You may recall that I had discussed that low thyroid function is a cause of elevated cholesterol. Lowering cholesterol levels with statins can adversely affect the production of sex hormones. People with low thyroid function also have adrenal dysfunction. In essence, there is no such thing as a single hormone deficiency. He complained of chronic fatigue, not sleeping well, soreness after workouts to the point he avoided further physical activity for days, and loss of libido with premature ejaculation.

He further reported a history of diverticulitis and reoccurring sinus infections. He brought in recent blood work that revealed his total cholesterol levels were 145 mg/dl (too low), reference range of 125-200 mg/dl, and TSH was 3.26 mIU/L (reference range .45-4.5 mIU/L). You may recall that I discussed that any readings of TSH over 2.0 m IU/L were suspect for hypo-function. I had the patient take his basal body temperature for five mornings, and it averaged 96.9, confirming under-function of the thyroid. The patient reported he was taking a synthetic one-a-day vitamin, fish oil capsules, and oral DHEA.

My initial impression was that this patient was still hypothyroid (probably a poor convertor of T4 to T3 because he felt no symptomatic improvement after he was started on the Levothyroxine), had adrenal dysfunction affecting cortisol levels, and all his hormone were probably low due to the low thyroid function. A saliva test was ordered and obtained, and then he was placed on a supplement providing the nutrients his body required to convert the Levothyroxine to T3, a nutraceutical for adrenal support, and sublingual liquid B Vitamins to help increase his energy levels during the day. When supporting a low thyroid, it is always necessary to support the adrenals. Two weeks later, he returned to go over his test results. See the test results below.

One of the unforeseen findings was an elevated progesterone level of over 6,000 pg/ml. This level was outside testing range for a man and could only come from contamination from a female who was using transdermal progesterone. Cross contamination can occur between sexual partners if an application of a hormone occurs just prior to coitus, in this case between the wife (not my patient) and the husband (my patient). Physical contact should be avoided for at least 15 minutes after application to allow absorption of the hormone. I provide this instruction to all my patients. The potential for long-term exposure of excess progesterone is feminization. This patient, however, did not exhibit any signs of gynecomastia or rounding of the hips or thighs. Estradiol and estrone levels were slightly elevated and testosterone levels were low at 94.5 pg/ml (reference range 130-135 pg/ml). His DHEA levels were high from the oral dosing, but he

Miller Clinic for Optimal Health - SALIVARY BIOLOGICAL TEST REPORT

Report Date: 7/9/2014
Date Received: 7/7/2014
Submitter Information
Institute: Miller Clinic for Optimal Health
Address: 11804A North 56th Street
Temple Terrace, FL 33617
Physician: Dr. Kelly Miller
Phone:

Patient Information
Name: BM
Date of Birth: 11/15/1961
Sex: M
Sample Collection Date: 6/24/2014
Sample ID No.: 14-00596

Last Menstrual Cycle: NA
Age of Menopause:
Hx of Surgery:
Medications: Levothyroxine
Send Lab Results To: Dr. Kelly Miller

HORMONE	LAB RESULT		FEMALE RANGE REFERENCE RANGE	FEMALE RANGE ASSESSED OPTIMUM RANGE WITH SUPPLEMENT	FEMALE RANGE ASSESSED OPTIMUM RANGE WITH TRANSDERMAL	MALE RANGE REFERENCE RANGE	MALE RANGE ASSESSED OPTIMUM RANGE WITH SUPPLEMENT	MALE RANGE ASSESSED OPTIMUM RANGE WITH TRANSDERMAL	Recommendation
Progesterone pg/ml Reportable Range 10-6900 pg/mL	>6,000	Follicular 1/14 days	28-82	100-2500	200-5000	<26	20-100	200-2500	
		Luteal 15/28 days	127-446						
		Post Menopause	18-51						
Estrone pg/mL Reportable Range 1.4 - 300 pg/mL	<1.4		3-20	N/A	N/A	3-6	N/A	N/A	
Estradiol pg/ml Reportable Range 1.3-300 pg/mL	4.3	Follicular	5-9	10-20	20-100	<2.5	N/A	N/A	
		Peak Max	12-20	10-20	20-100				
		Luteal	3-7	10-20	20-100				
		Post Menopause	1.5-3	10-20	20-100				
Estriol pg/ml Reportable Range 1.0-1200 pg/mL	NA		2-25	10-50	20-250	NA	NA	NA	
RATIO	NA	Progesterone/Estradiol	Optimum Ratio of Progesterone / Estradiol ≥ 20 (For Female only)						
RATIO	NA	Estriol/Estradiol	Optimum Ratio of Estriol / Estradiol ≥ 4 (For Female only)						
Testosterone pg/ml Reportable Range 8.2 - 2000 pg/mL	94.5	AGE 20-29 30-39 40-49 50-59 60-69	45-49 40-45 35-40 30-35 25-30	40-60 40-60 40-60 40-60 40-60	100-300 100-300 100-300 100-300 100-300	145-155 140-145 135-140 130-135 125-130	140-165 140-145 140-165 140-165 140-165	250-2000 250-2000 250-2000 250-2000 250-2000	
DHEA pg/ml Reportable Range 1.0-2000 pg/ml	776.3	AGE 20-29 30-39 40-49 50-59 60-69 70-79 Over 80	270-300 240-270 210-240 180-210 150-180 120-150 80-120	250-300 250-300 250-300 250-300 250-300 250-300 250-300	300-3000 300-3000 300-3000 300-3000 300-3000 300-3000 300-3000	300-330 270-300 240-270 210-240 180-210 150-180 100-150	300-350 300-350 300-350 300-350 300-350 300-350 300-350	350-3500 350-3500 350-3500 350-3500 350-3500 350-3500 350-3500	
CORTISOL nmol/L Reportable Range 0.09-158 nmol/L			ASSESSED OPTIMUM RANGE				ASSESSED OPTIMUM RANGE		
1st hour	6.43		13-18				13-18		
4th hour			6-9				6-9		
7th hour			3-6				3-6		
10th hour			2-3				2-3		
13th hour	4.47		1-2				1-2		

STOP SUPPLEMENT 24 HRS. PRIOR TO SALIVA SAMPLE

was not converting it to testosterone. He was converting most of it to androstenedione and then to estrone. His cortisol levels were very low at 6.43 mmol/L (reference range 13-18 mmol/L, ideal 16-18mmol/L). This cortisol level confirmed adrenal dysfunction, which always accompanies a hypothyroid condition.

To repair these conditions, the patient was placed on natural aromatase inhibitors to encourage more conversion of DHEA to testosterone and discourage the conversion of androstenedione to estrone and testosterone to estradiol. He was instructed to avoid further progesterone contamination and given a transdermal enzyme that helped convert the progesterone into testosterone. He was also given a nutraceutical that would increase his endogenous production of testosterone by about fifty percent. He was switched from oral DHEA to transdermal DHEA to reduce liver stress. In addition, I recommended a blend of three types of cordycep mushrooms to detoxify his liver and improve the H-P-A, H-P-T, and H-P-G axis. The supplements previously recommended for the conversion of T4 to T3, adrenal support, and B Vitamins were continued.

Four weeks later, B. M. was seen for a follow-up evaluation. He reported that his energy level was up, that he was sleeping better, and now was able to workout three times per week without muscle soreness. In addition, he felt that his muscle mass and tone had improved, he had lost five pounds, and his love life was better. I recommended that he continue his current dosing for two more months and be re-tested for fine tuning of the supplementation.

This case particularly demonstrates that there is no such thing as a single hormone deficiency. It also demonstrates that the conversion of synthetic T4 drugs like Levothyroxine often does not occur into the more bio-active form of T3 and that adrenal dysfunction always accompanies a hypothyroid condition. The Levothyroxine did not address all his hormone deficiencies. His low thyroid function probably played a role in his original diagnosis of elevated cholesterol of 220 mg/dl ten years ago.

Take the thyroid self-assessment to help determine if your thyroid function is optimum.

THYROID SELF-ASSESSMENT [1]
(Used with permission of author)

Thyroid Deficiency
If supplementation has begun, increase dosage.

Excessive coldness
Fatigue

Thinning skin
Weight gain
Dry skin and hair
Chronic constipation
Thinning hair and eyebrows
Mental dullness

Thyroid Excess
If supplementation has begun, decrease dosage.

Anxiousness
Weight los despite increased caloric intake
Trembling
Shaky hands
Intense sweating

Chapter 15 References

1. Tai PL. *8 Powerful Secrets to Anti-Aging.* Dearborn Heights, MI: Health Secrets, USA; 2007.
2. Tai PL. *Clinical Nutrition.* Dearborn Heights, MI: Health Secrets USA; pending publication.
3. Barnes BO. *Hypothyroidism: The Unsuspected Illness.* Trumbull, CT: Broda O Barnes, MD, Research FD; 1976.
4. Brownstein D. *Overcoming Thyroid Disorders.* West Bloomfield, MI: Medical Alternatives Press; 2008.
5. Brownstein D. *Iodine: Why You Need It, Why You Can't Live Without It.* West Bloomfield, MI: Medical Alternatives Press; 2009.

Chapter 16: Melatonin

Melatonin is known by most people for its ability to help jet lag or insomnia,[1-3] but the reality is it has many other functions in the body. It is the most powerful anti-oxidant found to date.[1-4] It is also important in our sense of well being and is associated with longevity.[1-3] Melatonin is the oldest of all the hormones, probably over three billion years old. Produced by the pineal gland in humans, it is found in algae, in every plant, and in every animal on the planet.[5-6] Exposing the eyes to bright sunlight stimulates the production of serotonin during the day and melatonin during the night. Melatonin is produced best in total darkness and is responsible for our sleep/wake cycle.

This amazing hormone assists and enhances the immune system, is involved in the production of growth hormone, improves mood, helps the response to stress, decreases and modulates cortisol, is a powerful anti-oxidant, stimulates the release of the sex hormones, stimulates the parathyroid for bone formation, and prevents cancer in several ways by inhibiting cell proliferation and helping to facilitate cellular death (apoptosis).[1,4,7] Cells are programmed to die after 7, 30, 60, or 120 days, depending on the type of cell. It is a powerful antioxidant. If you are experiencing light, anxious or agitated sleep, are easily awakened, have difficulty falling back to sleep, have poor dreaming, hypersensitivity and irritability, you might have melatonin deficiency.[1]

Arnold Lerner, M.D., began researching melatonin in 1953. He was trying to find a way to lighten skin color.[8] While he was not successful in finding a way to lighten the skin with melatonin, he did discover other functions for melatonin, one of them being that there seemed to be no side effects or toxicity, other than mild sedation for some subjects, even when he was injecting up to 200 mg into his subjects by 1960.[3] Additionally, melatonin supplementation has proven effective in sleep disorders in general,[9, 10] sleep disorders in blind people,[11] sleep disorders in autism[12-13] and mental retardation,[11] to improve symptoms of jet lag,[14-15] insomnia,[11] and improving the effectiveness of certain cancer medications.[16-17] It decreases the symptoms of *TD* (tardive dyskinesia), treats cluster headaches, and reduces anxiety.[1,3,9]

Melatonin levels rise from birth till about one year of age and, then, are fairly constant till puberty. During puberty, a drop in melatonin signals estrogen production, which in turn stimulates estrogen receptors in the bones to close the epiphysis (growth plate). Children who have higher levels of melatonin reach an older age before puberty begins and, therefore, have more height potential. Children who reach puberty at an early age have been shown to have melatonin levels at one-third of average. Melatonin levels start to decline in middle to older age.[18]

Is it possible that the reason that women live longer than men is because women have higher melatonin levels than men?[19-22] Four studies done in France, Switzerland, and Germany suggest so. In each of the studies, women tested anywhere from twenty to thirty percent higher in melatonin levels compared to men of the same age. There have also been studies comparing an elderly population of healthy seniors vs. senile seniors of the same age, and the healthy seniors had higher melatonin levels compared to the senile group. A 1993 Italian study showed a clear correlation between mental acuity in the elderly and melatonin levels. The healthy elderly had over two times higher melatonin levels compared to individuals of the same age who had been diagnosed with Alzheimer's disease.[19] Alzheimer's patients have demonstrated high levels of free radicals in brain. Most knowledgeable nutritionists will tell you that the three most powerful antioxidants are *superoxide dismutase, catalase* and *glutathione*. However, melatonin is five times more powerful than glutathione.[1] It may be that higher levels of melatonin give protection from free radicals in the brain and the development of Alzheimer's.

In 1985, George Maestroni found evidence of melatonin's ability to extend life.[23] His study was with two groups of mice. One group was given plain water, and the other group was given water with melatonin added. The mice group receiving plain water lived for 752 days on average, and the group with the melatonin lived for 931 days on average, or twenty percent longer. Another study was conducted in 1998 with rats.[24] After fifteen months, eighty-seven percent of the rats receiving melatonin were still alive while only forty-three percent of the rats without melatonin were still living. Of the seven rats left surviving in the control group without melatonin supplementation, five had pneumonia. Conversely, all the rats in the group treated with melatonin showed no signs of illness.

You are probably thinking that is all well and good the mice and rats, but what about us humans? A study of twenty-three centenarians demonstrated that they had higher levels of melatonin than the people in that control group that were only fifty to sixty years of age.[23] At this point, if you are like me, you want to know how you can maximize and preserve your melatonin levels. Am I right?

In 1993, there was an important study of fifteen men and women in their twenties to thirties who were exposed to bright light for four hours each day for two days vs. a similar demographic group that was not exposed to any bright light during this time. After two days, the two groups were tested. The group that was exposed to the bright light for four hours scored significantly better in cognitive functions, wakefulness, reaction times, and sense of well-being.[26] From other research, we now know that at least one hour of bright sunlight is needed to properly stimulate the hypothalamus, which in turn signals the pineal gland, to produce adequate amounts of melatonin. More sunlight is better. So you see, not only does sunlight stimulate the production of Vitamin D through our skin, but it also stimulates the production of melatonin through our eyes.

However, for our bodies to produce melatonin at optimal levels requires total darkness at night. Make sure no light is coming through your windows in your bedroom. Shut off your electronics that have lights at night. Do not go into the bathroom or kitchen and turn on the light in the middle of the night. If you do, you will shut down your melatonin production. You should also not have bright lights on after dark. Melatonin is very sensitive to certain wavelengths of light, especially from 460-480 angstroms. This is known as blue light, the kind of light your computer screen emits. Turn your computer off after dark. In fact, bright light at night is detrimental to your health.

The International Agency for Cancer Research has classified lights at night as a group 2B carcinogen.[27] The cancer rate for large metropolitan populations is much higher when compared to rural areas. New York, London, Paris, Chicago, and other large cities have significantly higher cancer rates compared to small towns and rural areas in close proximity. Those cities that are farther away from the equator also have higher cancer rates. Can you guess why? They are farther away from the proper angle of the sunlight through the winter months that allows for Vitamin D production in the skin, causing Vitamin D levels to be lower during winter months. I discuss Vitamin D later in the book. Both melatonin and Vitamin D are master hormones in the body.

The less sleep you get the less melatonin you produce. People who sleep six hours or less have an increased mortality rate of seventy percent compared to those who sleep seven to eight hours. Proper sleep is critical to health and well-being. In a study of twenty-four healthy men who agreed to be awakened at 3:00 AM and not allowed to return to sleep, a reduction of twenty-five percent of the body's own *natural killer* cells was demonstrated.[15] Natural killer cells are part of the immune system that identify and eliminate cancer cells in the body. It did not take weeks or months for this deficiency to occur. It only took one day. People who work the night shift have higher cancer rates than the same employees of the same age, doing the same job, only on a day shift. We are not designed to be awake in bright lights in the wee hours of the morning.

Insomnia is a fairly common complaint. Unfortunately, both prescription and nonprescription sleep aids cause marked melatonin suppression. Drugs like Halcion and Valium, which are commonly prescribed for depression and anxiety, also inhibit melatonin production.[28-29] The simple and no-side-effects solution is to take melatonin if you need help to sleep. There are a few other common medications, such as aspirin, ibuprofen, (less so with Tylenol),[30-31] pain medications, *beta-blockers*,[31-32] steroids, coffee at night, and tobacco that inhibit melatonin. Another offender is EMFs (electromagnetic frequencies).[37] A study of women using an electric blanket at night found it caused a seventy-five percent suppression of melatonin production.[9] Because of this it would be a good idea to keep all electrical devices that are turned on at night several feet away from where you sleep.

A 1993 M.I.T. study showed even small amounts of supplemental melatonin allowed people to relax, get to sleep faster, and stay asleep longer.[38] In addition to the hour of sunlight in our eyes mentioned earlier, there are other natural ways to stimulate your melatonin production. One method is to increase core temperature by a couple of degrees by getting into a sauna, hot tub, or just a hot bath or shower before going to bed. *Tryptophan, St. John's Wort*, and prayer (meditation) all increase your melatonin as well.[39]

Melatonin has shown promise in the treatment of pain. There was a large study of depressed individuals vs. those in chronic pain.[21] The study was done because apparently there were several similarities in the hormone patterns of these two groups. The

---

124

interesting thing to me about this study is that forty-four percent of the chronic pain patients noted marked improvement in their physical discomfort with melatonin supplementation. This is significant because for those people who do not suffer from depression before the development of the chronic pain, when the pain leaves so does the depression. Further studies with mice showed that melatonin's effectiveness for pain was dose dependent. Dose for dose, melatonin was found just as effective as morphine in reducing adverse reaction to pain in the mice.[21]

Melatonin may create a sense of well-being.[1-3] We do not yet know the full extent of involvement of melatonin, but it is interesting to note that in a manic-depressant individual the melatonin levels are two times higher than normal in the manic phase, and melatonin levels are below normal in the depressed phase.[11] In a 1992 study of schizophrenic patients, subnormal levels of melatonin were noted. When surgeons have had to remove the pineal gland due to brain cancer, people suffer from depression, anxiety, excessive sleepiness, headaches, auditory, and visual hallucination-- similar to the symptoms of schizophrenia.[40] Autism is another complex neurological problem. One of the observations made was that these children do not have a natural surge of melatonin at night.[12] Most of these children have difficulty sleeping, and melatonin supplementation is effective for this.

Melatonin levels in the body may play a role in cancer rates. Breast cancer is five times more common in industrialized countries than in developing nations, but fifty percent of the reason for this is currently unaccounted for. However, women who work the night shift have an increased breast cancer incidence.[41-43] Working at night inhibits melatonin production, and physiological levels of melatonin inhibit breast cancer cell proliferation. Studies using melatonin coupled with the chemotherapy drug, Tomaxifen, proved to be sixty percent more effective than Tomaxifen alone.[41-44] To create this effect, the melatonin had to be administered at night.

Each year two hundred thousand new cases of prostate cancer are diagnosed with a forty thousand per year annual mortality rate. If the cancer is found when it is localized, there is a seventy-five percent survival rate over five years. Supplemental melatonin has been shown to inhibit prostate cancer cell proliferation.[12] Melatonin has been very effective in protecting bone marrow

125

from damage from chemotherapy. Melatonin also inhibits breast, prostate, lung, and liver cancer and protects against radiation.[45]

In summary, melatonin seems to be necessary for a good sense of well-being. It is essential to our natural *bio-circadian* cycles and sleep/wake cycle. It is the most powerful antioxidant known to man, attacking free radicals. It has amazing characteristics for cancer protection, gives protection to our brain, and seems to be related to our longevity.

As a physician specializing in Aging and Regenerative Medicine, I am very excited about what melatonin can do for my patients and for me. For all of the above reasons, I personally use two grams of transdermal melatonin, rubbing it into my face every night before going to bed. No long term negative side effects have ever been documented, and supplementation does not affect your body's own production of melatonin.

Take the melatonin self-assessment to help determine if your body is producing optimal melatonin levels.

MELATONIN SELF-ASSESSMENT [1]
(Used with permission of author)

Melatonin Deficiency	Melatonin Excess
If supplementation has begun, increase dosage.	If supplementation has begun, decrease dosage.
Insomnia	Sleepy, groggy after working
Inability to stay awake	Inability to wake
Walking periodically throughout the night	Recurring nightmares or unpleasant dreams
Jet lag	Daytime sleepiness, fatigue
Difficulty adjusting to new time zones	Depressed, craving for sugar
Headaches	Increased cortisol and fat
Headaches	

Chapter 16 References

1. Tai PL. *8 Powerful Secrets to Anti- Aging*. Dearborn Heights, MI: Health Secrets USA; 2007
2. Dahlitz M, Alvarez B, Vignau J, et al. Delayed sleep phase syndrome response to melatonin. *Lancet* 1991 May 11; 337(8750): 1121-4.
3. Oldani A, Ferini-Strambi L, Zucconi M, Stankov B, Fraschini F, Smime S. Melatonin: delayed sleep and phase syndrome; ambulatory polygraphic evaluation. *Neuro Report,* 1994; 6:132-134.
4. Bland J. *Obesity and Endocrine signaling*. Health Com. International, Inc.; 1999.
5. Kolaf J, Machaackova I. Melatonin: Does it Regulate Rhythmicity and Photoperiodism Also in Higher Plants? *Flowering Newsletter* 1994; (17): 53.
6. Pieggeier B. Melatonin as the Light-Dark Zertgeber in Vertebrates, Invertebrates, and Unicellular organisms. *Experimentia* 1993; 49: 611-613.
7. Lieberman, S. *The Real Vitamin and Mineral Book*. New York: Avert Publ.; 1997.
8. Lerner AB, Case JD, Takahashi Y, Lee TH, Mori W. Isolation of Melatonin, the Pineal Gland Factor that Lightens Melanocytes. *J Am Chem Soc* 1958. 80910): 2587-2587. DOI: 10.1021/ja01543a060
9. Duell PB, Wheaton DL, Shultz A, Nguyen H. Inhibition of LDL oxidation by melatonin requires supraphysiologic concentrations. *Clin Chem* 1998; 44(a); 1931-1936.
10. Tan, DX, Manchester LC, Reiter RJ, et al. A novel melatonin metabolite, cyclic-3- hydroxymelatonin, a bio-marker of in vivo hydroxyl radical generation. *Biochem Biophys Res Commun* 1998 Dec 30; 253(30: 614-20.
11. Clainstrat B, Brun J, Chazot G. Melatonin in Humans, Neuroendocrinological and Pharmacological Aspects. *Int J Rad Apple Instrum B* 1990: 17(7): 625-32.
12. Loeb S, ed. *Professional Guide to Diseases, 4th Ed.* Springhouse, PA: Springhouse Corp. 1992.
13. Kielmann G, Neri F, Lissoni P. Lack of Light/Dark rhythm of the Pineal Hormone Melatonin (MLT) in

Autistic Children,. Presented at the First International Congress of Clinical Neuromodulation. Monza, Italy. 1995.

14. Parry BL, Berga SL, Kripke DF, Gillan JC. Melatonin and Phototherapy in Premenstrual Depression. *Prog Clin Biol Res* 1990; 341B: 35-43.

15. Irwin M, Mascovick A, Gillin JC, et al. Partial Sleep Deprivation Reduces Natural Killer Cells in Humans. *Psychosomatic Medicine* 1994; 56(6): 493-98.

16. Lissoni P, Barni S, Brivio F, Maestroni G. A Randomized Study with Sub-Cutaneous Low-Dose Interleukin 2 Alone Vs. Interleukin 2 Plus the Pineal Neurohormone Melatonin in Advanced Stage Neoplasms Other Than Renal Cancer and Melanoma. *British Journal of Cancer* 1994; 69: 196-99.

17. Lissoni P, Barni S, Brivio F, Maestroni G. Clinical Study Of Melatonin in Untreatable Advanced Cancer Patients. *Tumori* 1987; 73: 475-80.

18. Arendt J. Melatonin and the Pineal Gland; Influence of Mammalian Seasonal and Circadian Physiology. *Reviews of Reproduction* 1998; 3: 13-22.

19. Magnani M, Accorsi A. The Female Longevity Phenomenon: Hypothesis on Some Molecular and Cell Biology Aspects. *Mechanisms of Aging and Development* 1993; 72: 89-95.

20. Touitou Y, Fevre-Montagne M, NaKache JP. Age and Sex-Associated Modification of Plasma Melatonin Concentrations in Man's Relationship to Pathology (Malignant or Not) and Autopsy Findings. *Acta Endocrinologica* 1985; 108; 135-144.

21. Almay BGL, Von Knorring L, Wetterberg L. Melatonin in Serum and Urine in Patients with Idiopathic Pain Syndrome. *Psychiatry Research* 1987; 22: 179-91.

22. Birau N. Melatonin in Human Serum: Progress in Screening and Clinic. (Institute of Preventive Endocrinology, Bremen, Federal – Republic of Germany, 1980).

23. Maestroni G, Conti A, Pujaolih W. Pineal Melatonin: Its Fundamental Immunoregulatory Role, Aging and Cancer.

Annals of the New York Academy of Science 1988: 521: 140-148.

24. Oaknin-Bendahan S. Effects of Long-Term Administration of Melatonin and a Pulsatile Antagonist on the Ageing Rat. *Neuro Repor*, 1995; 6: 785-798.

25. Magri M, Sarra S, Chinetti W, et al. Qualitative and quantitative changes of melatonin levels in physiological and pathological aging and in centenarians. *Journal of Pineal Research* 2004 May; 36(4): 256-61.

26. Grinberger J, Linzmayer L, Saleta B. The Effect of Biologically-Active Light in the Noo- and Thymopsyche and on Psychophysiological Variables in Healthy Volunteers. *Int J Psychophysiol* 1993 July; 15(1): 27-37.

27. American Cancer Society. Known and Probably Human Carcinogens. www.cancer.org. Accessed June 1, 2016.

28. McIntyre I, Burrows GD, Norman TR. Suppression of Plasma Melatonin by a Single Dose of Benzodiazepine Alprozalam in Humans. *Biology Psychiatry* 1988; 24: 105-108.

29. Monteleone P, Farziati M, Maj M. Preliminary Observation in the Suppression of Nocturnal Plasma Melatonin Levels by Short-Term Administration of Diazepine in Humans. *Bilogical* 1988; 24: 105-108.

30. Murphy PJ, Badia P, Myers BL, Wright KP. Non-steroidal Anti-inflammatory Drugs Affect Normal Sleep Patterns in Humans. *Physiology and Behavior* 1994; 55(6): 1063-66.

31. Long JW, Rybacki J. *The Essential Guide to Prescription Drugs*. 1995. New York: Harper Perennial, 1995.

32. Brismar K, Hylander B, Wetterberg L. Melatonin Secretion Related to Side-Effects of Beta- Blockers from the Central Nervous System. *Acta Medica Scandinavia* 1988; 223: 525-30.

33. Wright KP, Badia P, Myers BL, Hakel M. Effects of Caffeine, Bright Light, and Their Combibation on Nighttime Melatonin and Temperature during Two Nights of Sleep Deprivation. *Sleep Research* 1995; 24: 458.

34. Wright KP, Badia P, Myers BL, Hakel M. The Combined Effects of Bright Light and Caffeine on Nighttime Alertness and Performance during Two Nights of Sleep Deprivation. *Sleep Research* 1995; 24: 459.

35. Wright KP, Badia P, Meyers BL, Hakel M. The Combined Effects of Bright Light and Caffeine on Nighttime Melatonin during Two Nights of Sleep Deprivation. *Sleep Researc.* 1995; 24: 460.

36. Doll R, Peto R, Boreham J, Sutherland I. Mortality in Relation to Smoking: 50 Years Observations in Male British Doctors. *British Medical Journal* 1994; Oct 8; 309(6959): 901-11.

37. Willson BW, Wright KP, Anderson LE. Evidence for an effect of ELF Electromagnetic Fields on Human Pineal Gland Function. *Journal of Pineal Research* 1990; 9: 259-69.

38. Dollins AB, Wurtman RJ, Deng MH. Effect of inducing Nocturnal Serum Melatonin Concentration in Daytime on Sleep, Mood, and Body Temperature, and Performance. Proceedings of the *National Academy of Science* 1994; 91: 1824-28.

39. Masscon AO, Tear J, Katat-Zimu J. Meditation, Melatonin, and Breast/Prostate Cancer: Hypothesis and Preliminary Data. *Medical Hypothesis* 1995; 44: 39-46.

40. Monteleone P, Maj M, Fusco M, Kemali D, Reiter RJ. Depressed Nocturnal Plasma Melatonin Levels in Drug-Free Paranoid Schizophrenics. *Schizophrenia Research* 1992; 7: 77-84.

41. Lissoni P, Barni S, Meregalli S, Fossati V, Cazzaniga M, Esposti D, Tancini G. Modulation of cancer endocrine therapy by melatonin: a phase II study of tamoxifen plus melatonin in metastatic breast cancer progressing under tamoxifen alone. *British Journal of Cancer* 1995; 70: 001-003.

42. Blask DF, Hull SM. Effects of Melatonin in Cancer. Studies on MCF7 Human Breast Cancer Cells in Culture. *Journal of Neural Transmission* 1986; 28: 433-47.

43. Cos S, Sanchez-Barcelo E. Difference between Pulsatile or Continuous Exposure to Melatonin on MCF-7 Breast Cancer Cell Proliferation. *Cancer Letters* 1994; 85: 105-109.

44. Cos S, Blask DF, Hill SM. Effects of Melatonin in the Cell Cycle Kinetics and Estrogen Rescue of MCF-7

Human Breast Cancer Cells in Culture. *Journal of Pineal Research* 1991; 10: 36.

45. Vijayalaxmi BZ, Reiter RJ, Sewerynek E, Meltz L, Poeggler B. Melatonin Protects Human Blood Lymphocytes from Radiation Induced Chromosome Damage. *Mutation Researc. 1995; 346(1): 23.*

Chapter 17: Vitamin D

You may be wondering why I am writing about Vitamin D in a hormone book. The truth of the matter is that Vitamin D is not only a vitamin, but it is also a hormone. Vitamin D is manufactured when sunlight strikes the skin, and it then is converted from cholesterol. It is the daytime hormone that complements our nighttime hormone, melatonin. Both of these hormones are activated by sunlight.

Vitamin D has always been known for enhancing calcium along with phosphorous and magnesium absorption in the small intestines. In school thirty-something years ago, I was taught that if you had a Vitamin D deficiency you had *rickets disease* (a bone deformity illness). Very few people had rickets by 1980, so it was felt that nobody had Vitamin D deficiency problems. Also, there was a lot of fear of overdosing on Vitamin D at this time although it was unfounded. To put this into a context you can better understand, rickets disease is the end result of a severe Vitamin D deficiency, just as a goiter is the end result of a severe iodine deficiency. However, because we don't have rickets, does not mean we don't necessarily have a problem with a Vitamin D deficiency.

Scurvy was a common problem among sailors undertaking long voyages. It was eventually discovered that if the sailors ate limes or potatoes, they did not get scurvy because these two foods provided enough Vitamin C to prevent this disease from occurring. Because we don't have scurvy anymore does not mean we don't necessarily have a Vitamin C deficiency. These pathologies— rickets, goiter, and scurvy—are examples of what happens to our physiology when these deficiencies are extreme.

Vitamin D is responsible for over one hundred-fifty biological functions.[1,2] It is in control of over two hundred genes. To get adequate Vitamin D, we need to have total body exposure to the sun for about an hour and to be south of the northern border of Texas during the winter months to get sunlight at the proper angle from November to February.[3] This amount of exposure provides the average person with about 10,000 IU/day of Vitamin D. How many of you who do live south of the northern border of Texas are going nude in the sun for an hour every day? If you are one of these individuals, you don't need to read any further. You are probably OK.

It is interesting to note that I moved to Tampa, Florida, in

October 2013. Since that time I have evaluated many patients, routinely checking Vitamin D levels. The highest reading I have seen on a new patient is a level of 36 ng/ml. Reference ranges in most labs now run about 30-100 ng/ml for Vitamin D levels. Most of the patients that I have evaluated had Vitamin D levels in the twenties, and this is in Florida, the "Sunshine State".

Like all other hormones, it is better to be in the upper quartile (25%) of a reference range vs. the lower quartile (25%). In fact, if your Vitamin D levels 25 (OH) D levels) are under 19.7 mg/ml, you have an independent risk factor for all mortality.[4-6] You are more likely to die of a heart attack, stroke, cancer, diabetes, kidney disease autoimmune disease, Alzheimer's, and other degenerative diseases. Conversely, people in the upper quartile (25%) have three to four hundred percent less incidence of many diseases than those in the lower quartile (25%) of reference range.[4-6] You want to be in the 80-100 ng/ml range for 25 (OH) D levels, in my opinion. Those individuals that live at the equator and are out in the sun all day have 25 (OH) D levels averaging 130 mg/ml. These levels are similar to the levels of 25(OH) D for primates that live near the equator.[8]

Vitamin D is anti-cancer, anti-heart attack, anti-diabetic, anti-autoimmune disease, anti-kidney disease, anti-depressant, and anti-anxiety.[1-11] If you have optimum levels of Vitamin D, your body can activate cells to produce broad-spectrum antibiotics and activate genes that produce natural anti-viral substances.

Every cell in your body has a receptor site for Vitamin D. When a cell has a receptor site for a hormone, it means that the function of that cell is dependent upon the binding of that hormone for the receptor. In other words, if there is not an adequate Vitamin D level in your body to bind with the receptors, the cells in your body cannot do what they were designed to do.

Since we are not getting sun due to limited skin exposure, and, because of the broad use of sunscreen, generally most of us are Vitamin D deficient. Most of us are not getting enough Vitamin D in our multi-vitamin, or by taking 1000-2000 IU/day as many doctors recommend. There is also a problem with many people absorbing vitamin D due to genetic variances or problems in the ileum of the small intestine. About half the population has difficulty absorbing oral Vitamin D supplement in pill form. Also, the darker your skin color the harder it is for the sunlight to make Vitamin D. Mexican Americans and African Americans tend to have lower levels of

Vitamin D compared to European American populations in the same geographic region.

Not all supplements are created equal. D3 is more readily absorbed when it is taken in conjunction with K2. The receptors sites are side by side in most cells. K2 is a form of Vitamin K that is essential in the bone matrix providing tensile strength, vs. K1, which is involved with blood clotting. Both Vitamin D and K2 reduce soft tissue calcification and encourage bone calcification. You get better absorption with a D3/K2 combination. Vitamin D is not a prescription drug. The 50,000 IU prescription you are getting from your MD is not what you need. This is a synthetic form of D2, made from radiating fungus and plant matter. Please take D3/K2, not D2 for best results. It has been shown an individual can take up to 40,000 IU/day without any toxicity. It has been my experience that many people need between 10,000-20,000IU/day to bring 25(0H) D to optimal levels.

Nearly forty percent of the American public suffers from some form of cardiovascular disease. The most significant cause of this is coronary artery disease. There are two types of plaquing that occur in the arteries, a calcified hard plaque and a soft plaque. The first kind of plaquing is from calcification indirectly related to your hormones. The second kind, soft plaque, is related to VLDL (super-small sticky cholesterol particles) and inflammation. The soft plaque is what causes the *sudden death* heart attack. Low Vitamin D levels increase PTH (parathyroid) activity, which increases coronary calcification. Low Vitamin D is associated with increased renal failure from increased arterial calcification and vascular events. Lower Vitamin D levels contribute to insulin resistance, affects renin, affects polymorphism (gene variants), create inflammatory cytokine, all of which are directly related to cardiovascular diseases. The higher the amount of Vitamin D in the 4th quartile has the lowest rate of morbidity.[3] The lowest quartile (25%) has the highest rate of morbidity. Vitamin D stimulates osteoblastic activity (new bone growth) and decreases osteoclastic activity (taking away old bone cells). Decreased Vitamin D levels increase inflammatory *cytokines, TNFa* and *IL-1* (all inflammatory markers for the cardiovascular system), and increases local calcification in the blood vessels.[10]

Lower Vitamin D levels increase the risk of hypertension (high blood pressure) by 560%. In a study of 30,000 men, it was found that the further away from the equator the men lived the higher the incidence of hypertension.[11] The higher the Vitamin D levels the less hypertension and less calcification. There is also better kidney function with higher levels of Vitamin D. Sunlight increases Vitamin D levels and is associated with lower systolic and decreased blood pressure.[11] The lower the Vitamin D levels, the higher the parathyroid function,[12] and increased risk of hypertension.[13]

There is an inverse relationship between myocardial infarction and Vitamin D levels.[14] There is a seasonality of cardiovascular mortality, most probably due to the protective effect of more ultraviolet radiation from the sun in summer months. In the winter months, we have more acute *myocardial infarction* (heart attacks). The less sunshine we get the less Vitamin D we make and the more occurrence of acute myocardial infarction (heart attack).[15]

Chronic heart failure is associated with reduced Vitamin D levels, which may result in a number of conditions: increased TNFa and pro-inflammatory cytokines (inflammatory markers that affect blood vessels), reduced myocardial compliance (resistance to filling), and contractility (output), increased PTH (parathyroid) and associated calcium metabolism affecting sodium channels, which may cause arrhythmias.[16,17] Vitamin D deficiency is also associated with increased risk of Diabetes type II and Syndrome X because both Diabetic type II and Syndrome X have an inverse correlation to vitamin D and calcium.[18] Syndrome X, also known as Metabolic Syndrome, is denoted by a clustering of three of five of the following conditions:

- central abdominal obesity,
- elevated blood pressure,
- elevated fasting plasma glucose,
- elevated serum triglycerides, and
- low high density lipoprotein (HDL) levels.

Vitamin D beta cell receptors regulate insulin response to glucose, improve insulin action at the receptor, improve glucose transport, help maintain extracellular calcium for membrane transports of glucose, and modulate inflammatory cytokines that increase *beta cell apoptosis,* and enhance cell regeneration.[13] Low Vitamin D levels increase insulin resistance and pancreatic beta cell dysfunction.[13] In effect optimum levels of Vitamin D make your insulin more effective at getting glucose (sugar) inside your cells to be used for energy and helps the beta cells that produce insulin to better function. Conversely, low levels of Vitamin D will cause insulin resistance and high blood sugars associated with Type II Diabetes and Syndrome X. As to be expected, *glycemic* (blood sugar) control is worse in the winter when most people get less sunlight.[13]

Vitamin D testing can be included whenever you get a blood panel ordered by your doctor. We do Vitamin D testing in the office using a dried blood spot test kit. It can also be done at home. You simply prick the end of a finger with a small lancet provided in the kit. Blood spot testing is actually more accurate than serum testing. The dried blood is analyzed with gas chromatography, which is considered the gold standard for blood analysis.

Because of the problems with so many people lacking the ability to properly absorb Vitamin D, we recommend a liquid sublingual D3/K2 form with liposome technology.[19] This is the best delivery system available today.

Estrogen, Progesterone, and Vitamin D Case History

B. S. was a sixty-one-year-old physical therapist who came in wanting testing for food/chemical allergy/sensitivity and saliva hormone testing due to her osteopenia. She had been on synthetic estrogen in the past for her bone density and oral natural progesterone, and she had some previous allergy testing. Her last allergy testing and bone density testing had been performed in 2012, two years prior. Her other chief concerns in addition to her allergies and osteopenia were that her energy was not as good as she wanted it to be, her sleep was often interrupted, she wanted to lose some weight and was having difficulty doing so, and she had mild to moderate intermittent joint pains.

The *MRT* (Mediator Release Test) for food/chemical allergy/sensitivity found she had severe reactions to celery and had moderate reactions to FD&C Red Dye, salicylic acid (aspirin), *ibupropen,* saccharine, sodium sulfite, FD& C Yellow #5, tryamine, yoghurt, basil, lemon, olive, grapefruit, cucumber, carrot, oat, millet, tuna, clam, pork, egg, tapioca, lentils, and cashews. I recommended that she avoid all foods/chemicals on her list for four weeks to reduce immune and/or inflammatory responses. The patient had been eating celery, cucumbers, and carrots three to four times a week along with oatmeal, tuna, egg, and was a frequent ibupropen user for her joint pain.

The significance of food/chemical allergy/sensitivity is that they cause inflammation, which causes the adrenals to work harder to produce more cortisol, encouraging more body fat deposits and discouraging muscle and bone development. Chronic inflammation causes chronic cortisol production that reduces DHEA and testosterone production, two anabolic hormones needed for tissue repair, and fatigues the adrenal glands. Chronic inflammation is a stress that depletes the sex hormones. The inflammatory foods and chemicals can also lead to a *leaky gut*. This occurs when a person has too much emotional, chemical, or mechanical stress in his/her life.

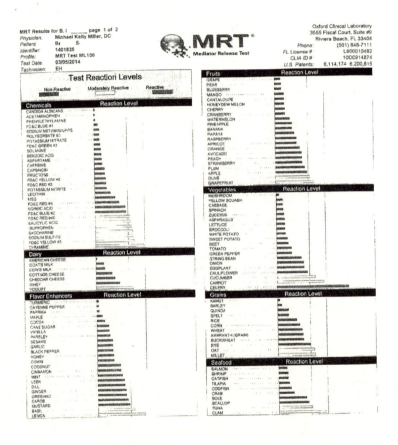

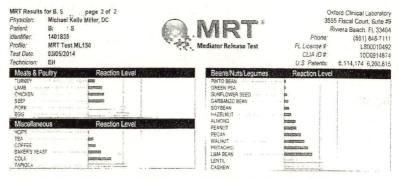

MRT Results for B. S   page 2 of 2
Physician: Michael Kelly Miller, DC
Patient: B   S
Identifier: 1401835
Profile: MRT Test ML150
Test Date: 03/05/2014
Technician: EH

Oxford Clinical Laboratory
3555 Fiscal Court, Suite #9
Riviera Beach, FL 33404
Phone: (561) 848-7111
FL License #:   L800010492
CLIA ID #:   10D0914674
U.S. Patents: 6,114,174 6,200,815

Meats & Poultry	Reaction Level
TURKEY	
LAMB	
CHICKEN	
BEEF	
PORK	
EGG	

Miscellaneous	Reaction Level
HOPS	
TEA	
COFFEE	
BAKER'S YEAST	
COLA	
TAPIOCA	

Beans/Nuts/Legumes	Reaction Level
PINTO BEAN	
GREEN PEA	
SUNFLOWER SEED	
GARBANZO BEAN	
SOYBEAN	
HAZELNUT	
ALMOND	
PEANUT	
PECAN	
WALNUT	
PISTACHIO	
LIMA BEAN	
LENTIL	
CASHEW	

Degrees of reactivity may not in all cases correlate with presence or level of clinical sensitivity to the food. Strongly positive results have been found to correlate with food reactivity. It is appropriate to eliminate foods with Reactive Scores. Moderately reactive scores should be evaluated by the physician or dietitian based upon patient history and frequency of consumption. After an appropriate period of elimination, reintroduce them one at the time under physician and/or dietitian supervision.
If negative foods have been consumed regularly before drawing the blood for the test, there is high probability that they are 'safe' and are not likely to provoke symptoms. If test positive foods are eliminated from the diet, these non-reactive foods reasonably could remain in the permitted diet during the elimination phase. The clinician or dietitian should remain alert to the possibility that any of these foods might provoke symptoms.

The test results of the saliva hormone test revealed extremely low levels of progesterone, estradiol, estriol, testosterone, and cortisol. DHEA levels were only slightly depressed. Estrone levels were elevated. You may recall that estrone levels follow body fat and there are two metabolites of estrone that are carcinogenic—16-alpha-hydroxyestrone and 4-hydroxyestrone. Elevated estrone levels without adequate B Vitamins for methylation of the metabolites and a deficiency of counter-balancing progesterone and estriol are a concern. I like to see a 20:1 progesterone/estradiol ratio and a 4:1 estriol/estradiol ratio in the post-menopausal woman for protection against estrogen related cancers. The progesterone and estriol help occupy receptor sites in the breast, uterus, and ovaries reducing the likelihood of a bad estrone metabolite landing there.

Sublingual liquid B Vitamins with liposome technology for methylation and a supplement containing I-3-C, DIM, chrysin, resveratrol, and peperine extract that encourages the production of more of the benign 2-hydroxyestrone metabolite. It was also important to have more progesterone available to stimulate new bone cells (*osteoblasts*) for the osteopenia. I advised transdermal progesterone and DHEA, and estradiol/estriol were recommended as well as an enzyme that converted her progesterone into testosterone. Balanced levels of estradiol/progesterone and DHEA and testosterone are necessary for good bone density. I also recommended a supplement containing nutrients and herbs for adrenal support with recommendations of getting to sleep by 10:00 PM and getting seven to eight hours of sleep.

Within two weeks B.S. reported her energy levels were better and she was sleeping better. She had lost five pounds. Her joint pain was mildly improved. On her next visit in two weeks she reported continued improvement in these same areas, but had some vaginal bleeding even though she had not had a cycle for over five years. (She actually called me about this.) This is a common temporary occurrence in some women starting progesterone. The reason this occurs is because there has been a build-up, a thickening of the uterus wall due to long-term estradiol excess with a progesterone deficiency.

Estradiol is a tissue builder in the first two weeks of the menstrual cycle. This is to prepare the uterus for pregnancy. If there is no conception, progesterone gets rid of the increased tissue growth during the menses. However, when a woman is progesterone deficient for many years an excess build-up of tissue occurs. This is why so many women have *fibroids* in the uterus, and this combination of excess buildup and progesterone deficiency is a contributing factor to *endometriosis*. Once a woman has adequate progesterone, the body gets rid of the excess. This is only a temporary inconvenience and should not be a cause for alarm. Progesterone supplementation cannot start your menstrual cycle once there are no more eggs. I assured her it would stop, and it did.

After three months of bio-identical and nutritional program, B.S. was re-tested. Her progesterone and estrogen levels had increased significantly, so her estradiol/estriol dosing was reduced. However, her DHEA, testosterone, and cortisol levels were still low. Her adrenal glands were still very fatigued and, therefore, were not producing adequate amounts of hormones. The adrenal cortex produces the cortisol as well as the DHEA and testosterone in the woman. Further inquiries revealed she was still working six days per week and staying up late on the computer. The adrenal glands just cannot repair without adequate rest. This is a common mistake too many of us make, and our health suffers. I re-emphasized that she needed more rest and increased dosing of transdermal DHEA and progesterone converter to testosterone was recommended. She finally decided to give up Saturday in her work schedule. I thanked her, and her adrenal glands thanked her.

After being on the bio-identical hormones and nutritional support, B.S. had a repeat bone density test done. Her bone density dramatically improved in her lumbar spine, with her going from a -1.0 to a -0.2. The Z-score represents her rating compared to other women her own age. Her *T-score* (bone density compared to an average 25-year-old) also improved, going from a -1.7 to a -1.0, which is considered normal by the World Health Organization. Bone density is not only dependent upon a proper balance of the sex hormones but is also dependent upon available Vitamin D. You may recall from the chapter on Vitamin D that there is an inverse relationship between Vitamin D and Vitamin K2 levels and bone density. This is why the combination of D3/K2 is more effective than D3 alone. On her last visit, she had lost an additional ten to fifteen pounds and looked great.

Chapter 17 References

1. Heaney RP, Reinhold R, Hollis BW. Vitamin D Efficacy and Safety. *Arch Intern Med* 2001; 171(3): 266. *doi: 10.1001/achinternmed.2010.528.*
2. Makariou S, Liberopoulos EN, Elisaf M, Challa A. Novel roles of Vitamin D inndisease: What is new in 2011? *European Journal of Internal Medicine* 201 August; 22(4): 355-362.
3. Watson KE, Abrolat ML, Malone LL, et al. Active Vitamin D levels are inversely associated with coronary calcification. *Circulation* 1997 Sept.16; 1197 (6): 1755-60
4. Dobnig H, Pilz S, Scharnagl H, et al. Independent Association of Low Serum 25-Hydroxyvitamin D and 1,25-Dihydroxyvitamin D levels With All-Cause and cardiovascular Mortality. *Arch Intern Med* 2008; 168(12): 1340-1349. *Doi: 10.1001/archinte.12.1340.*
5. Melamed ML, Michos ED, Post W, Astor B. 25-Hydroxyvitamin D Levels and the Risk of Mortality in the General Population. *Arch Intern Med* 2008; 168(15): 1629-1637.
6. Ginde AA, Scragg R, Schwartz RS, Camargo CA Jr. Vitamin D Supplementation and Total Mortality.: A Meat-Analysuis of Randomized Controlled Trials. *Arch*

Intern Med. 2007; 167(16); 1730-1737. *doi: 10.1001/archinte.167.16.1730.*

7. Grant WB. An estimate of the global reduction in mortality rates through doubling vitamin D levels. *European Journal of Clinical Nutrition* 20011; 65: 1016-1026. *doi: 10.1038/ejcn.2001.68; published online 6 July 2001.*

8. Adams JS, Chen H, Hun RF, et al. Novel regulators of Vitamin D action and metabolism: Lessons learned at the Los Angeles zoo. *Journal of Cellular Biochemistry*; 88(2): 308-314.

9. Tai PL. *8 Powerful Secrets of Anti-Aging.* Dearborn Heights, MI: Health Secrets USA; 2007.

10. Vimalieswaran KS, Cavadino A, Berry, DJ, et al. Association of vitamin D status with arterial blood pressure and hypertension risk: a mendelian randomization study. *Lancet Diabetes Endocrinol* 2014 Sep; 2(9): 719-29.

11. Reis, JP, von Muhlen D, Krist-Silverstein D, Wingard DL, Barrett-Connor E. Vitamin D, parathyroid hormone levels, and the prevalence of metabolic syndrome in community-dwelling older adults. *Eur J Endocrinol* 1994, 130; 446-450.

12. St John A, Dick I, Hoad K, Retallak R, Wellborn T, Prince R. Relationship between calcitrophic hormones and blood pressure in elderly subjects. *Eur J Endocrinol.* 1994, 130; 446-450.

13. Vitamin D receptor and prothrombotic factor. *J Biol Chem 2004.307 (suppl). 35798-35802*

14. Scragg E, Jackson R, Holdaway IA, Lim T, Beaglehole R. Myocardial Infarction is Inversely Associated with Plasm 2-Hydroxyvitamin D3 Levels: A Community-Based Study. *Inter J Epidemiol 1990 Sept. 29 (3):559-63*

15. Scragg R. Seasonality of cardiovascular disease mortality and the possible effect of ultra- violet radiation. *Inter J Epidemiol* 1981 Dec 1 (4): 337-41.

16. McCarty MF. Nutritional modulation of parathyroid hormone secretion may influence risk for left ventricular hypertrophy. *Med Hypothesis* 2005; 64 (30):1015-21.

17. Calcitriol modulation of cardiac contractile performance via protein Kinase C. *J. Mol. Cell Cardiol.* 2006 ;41.350-359

18. Chie KC, Chi, A, Vay LW, Go MF. Hypovitaminosis D is associated with insulin resistance and beta cell dysfunction. *Sci Acad Clin Nutr* 2004; 79:820-25.

19. El Asmar MS, Naoum JJ, Arbid EJ. Vitamin K dependent proteins and the role of vitamin K2 in the modulation of vascular calcification: a review. *Oman Med J* 2014 May; 29(3):172-7. *doi: 10.5001/omj.2014.44.*

Chapter 18: What Hormones We Test For

There are seven hormones evaluated in the women's saliva panel, including progesterone, estrone (EI), estradiol (E2), estriol (E3), testosterone, DHEA, and cortisol. Estriol is not evaluated in the men's panel as it does not occur in any abundance and no significant function has been determined in the physiology of men. Saliva samples are taken five times during the day, beginning within the first hour after waking and followed with approximately three-hour increments.

Progesterone levels are tested because this hormone gives protection to the breast, uterus, and ovaries. Progesterone converts to testosterone in men. Progesterone levels are highest in the last fourteen days of the menstrual cycle, and, generally speaking, symptoms occurring during this time are usually caused by a deficiency. Progesterone levels start to decline in women from age thirty to thirty-five.

Since estrone (E1) can form cancer-causing metabolites, such as 16-alpha-hydroxyestroe and 4-hydroxyestrone, it is important to test for this hormone as well. Excess levels increase the risk for breast, uterus, ovary, and prostate cancer. Estrone levels are fairly consistent with body fat levels. Estradiol (E2) is the abundant form of estrogen through the childbearing years and exists in a pool with estrone, interchanging as needed. Estradiol and progesterone give women cardiovascular protection in pre-menopause years. The final estrogen, estriol (E3) is the benign form of estrogen and gives protection to the breast, uterus, and ovaries. This form of estrogen cannot convert back to estrone or estradiol. Greatly increased levels of estriol during pregnancy gives added protection for the mother. For menopausal women, estriol alleviates hot flashes and vaginal dryness and helps sleep.

DHEA is an anabolic hormone, meaning it is important in the repair and building of tissue. It is important in cardiovascular health, immune system function, bone density, and reduces plaquing. People who live to be one hundred years of age or more have higher DHEA levels than those who are many years younger. Testosterone is necessary for bone and muscle development. It gives men and women confidence. It is important in reducing cardiovascular risk and is partially responsible for libido in both men and women. Finally, cortisol is necessary to make all cells work. It is out first hormonal line of defense against all stress and is involved in the fight or flight response. Furthermore, it is anti-inflammatory. Cortisol deficiencies are common after age forty.

These are the seven hormones that are evaluated in the saliva hormone panel. There are two other hormones, pregnenolone and the thyroid hormones, that are important for consideration that are not available to be tested in this panel. Pregnenolone is the precursor to both progesterone and DHEA. You may recall that progesterone converts to cortisol. Unfortunately, the pregnenolone molecule is not seen well in the saliva. However, diminished levels of DHEA, progesterone, and cortisol indicate a pregnenolone deficiency. Pregnenolone is very protective of the brain and nervous system.

Low thyroid hormones are a common cause of being overweight, obesity, fatigue, depression, mental fog, and infertility. Thyroid hormones are assessed with dried blood spot testing. IGF-1 can be assessed with dried blood spot testing as well.

Chapter 19: Different Testing Methods for Hormones

There are three ways to evaluate the hormones: through the blood, through the urine, and through the saliva. Each methodology has positive and negative outcomes. Blood testing is fairly straightforward. Almost everyone has had blood taken at one point in his/her life. You don't eat after midnight, and you show up at the lab first thing in the morning. All of us have done it. The sex hormones, growth hormone, thyroid hormones all can be evaluated through blood analysis. This is the most popular method for assessment that is used by doctors. There are several adverse circumstances associated with this methodology. The first is that some people are afraid of needles and, in fact, will faint at the sight of blood being drawn. The second is that this type of blood panel is expensive, costing $600 - $1,000 or more.

The third reason, and really the most significant for me, is that most of the hormones that are being evaluated are not bioactive. The vast majority of the hormone cannot be utilized by the receptors in any tissues because they are bound with something called SHGB, sex hormone binding globulin. In fact, ninety-five to ninety-eight percent of all hormones are bound by these substances. Only two to five percent are free, unbound, and available to attach to a waiting receptor site. To get a better idea of how much hormone is free, the doctor needs also to order a test for sex hormone-binding globulin and albumin. Many times the doctor does not order these additional tests, and the labs use arbitrary calculations to come up with the amount of free hormones. As a physician specializing in aging and regenerative medicine, I want to know exactly how much free hormone is available, not what is bound and on the way out of the body through the sweat, urine, or feces.

The second methodology for hormone analysis is through the urine. This is a very accurate form of assessment. It measures hormone levels by the many different metabolites that are in the urine. The cost of testing is much less, in the $300-$400 range, than blood analysis. One of the biggest drawbacks is that you have to keep all your urine in a container for a twenty-four hour period, keep it refrigerated, and get it to the lab afterwards. It is a bit of a hassle in my mind. More importantly, it does not accurately measure free hormones.

The third form of analysis of the sex hormones is through the

---

saliva. This is done by simply spitting into a straw, which then goes into a small tube. The tube is capped, and a small sticker is placed on it with the patient's name and date and time of collection. This is done within the first hour of waking and four more occasions throughout the day in approximately three-hour increments. The saliva is stable at room temperature for a few weeks. Moreover, the hormones that are measured are all free hormones because the sex hormone binding globulin molecule is too large to fit through the ducts in the month that produce saliva. The cost for a saliva sex hormone panel is under $300. To me, this method is head and shoulders above the other methods because it is extremely accurate, very easy to do, and the most cost effective as well. I would caution those who are using saliva testing as a diagnostic and monitoring tool if they are only taking one saliva reading each day. When done in this manner, it is no more accurate than a single serum blood hormone level is in determining total hormone output.

Chapter 20: Hormone Delivery Systems

There are several different ways doctors recommend administering hormones to their patients: injections, oral doses, surgically implanted pellets, and transdermal patches and creams. Before I get further into this discussion, I want to be perfectly clear about something. All three methods can be used for both synthetic and bio-identical hormones. I do not recommend the use of synthetic hormones as they have been shown to increase the risk of heart attacks, strokes, blood clots, and some cancers. If your doctor is prescribing synthetic hormones, I recommend finding another doctor who will use bio-identical hormones.

One method for administering hormones is through surgically implanted pellets. The only real advantage to this method is that the pellets last two to three months. There are, however, several unfavorable side effects. For one, you must go into the doctor's office for an outpatient surgical procedure. Your skin is cut open, which creates risk for infection. Sometimes the pellets come out through the skin. If the doctor does not get the dose correct, you can experience additional side effects, necessitating you to have to go back in the office to get the pellet removed and a different one inserted. The pellets usually deliver higher amounts initially, and then too little near the end. The only reason I can see this being done by a provider is that he or she can bill an insurance company for the surgical procedure and pellets.

The second method of delivery is through injections. When I initially started hormone therapy, my provider gave me a testosterone and a B12 shot every two weeks. I do not even like shots. The B12 shots were of *cyanocobalamin,* which is a form of B12 that cannot be used by the body. The cyanocobalamin has to be methylated, a (CH3+) molecule added, for the body to use this form of B12. The problem is that the process leaves a cyanide molecule in the body that has to be dealt with. When taking B12, only consume *methylcobalamin*, please. In addition to the inconvenience of having to go to the doctor's office every two weeks forever, the injection is a supra-physiological dose sometimes causing testosterone levels to spike above what the body deems normal.

This supra-physiological level triggers the liver to produce something called SHBG, which binds the testosterone and, unfortunately, every other sex hormone as the SHBG does not discriminate. The result of this is subpar hormone levels that stress the liver. A remedy for this by some doctors is have their patients come in two times each week for injections of smaller doses of hormone. I don't know about you, but I do not want to go to the doctor's office twice each week for the next thirty to forty years.

A third method of delivery is oral dosing by swallowing a pill or capsule. This method is fairly convenient and relatively inexpensive. However, there are a wide variety of absorption capabilities in the average population through the gastrointestinal tract. Many middle-aged and elderly people use over-the-counter and prescription antacids that inhibit the absorption of many nutrients and medications.

Also, *hypochlorhydria,* a decreased hydrochloric acid production, is common after the age of forty. If there is a deficiency in the stomach acid, there is also a deficiency in the pancreatic enzymes and bile secretion as it is the stomach acidity that triggers the enzymes and bile. Everything that goes into your mouth and into your stomach has to go through the liver before it passes through a cell membrane for use. If digestive capabilities are compromised sufficiently, then absorption is inhibited and hormone levels will not be at the desired level. On the other hand, if absorption is better than average, the dosing may be too high, causing supra-physiological levels to occur, activating liver production of SHBG. Also, some oral and sublingual forms irritate the tongue and gums.

While patches are fairly convenient, some people react to adhesive, causing rashes. By far, the most common method of delivery is by transdermal creams or lotions. Patches and creams account for seventy percent of the total application in use. There are many advantages to using transdermal creams. The first is that the specific type of hormone can be applied at the time of day that it naturally peaks. An example of this is applying transdermal testosterone first thing in the morning as this is the time that testosterone is at its highest level. This allows for better simulation of the natural circadian rhythms of a hormone. The transdermal hormone creams can be combined and compounded by a pharmacist requiring a doctor's prescription, or the individual hormone can be obtained, usually in a premeasured pump form.

One downside of a multi-hormonal compound is that if the level of just one of the hormones is too high or too low the whole formula had to be redone. The upside for a single hormone dispensed is that the dosage can be increased or decreased on a daily basis as needed. Transdermal methods have the advantage of the hormone being carried through the skin via the capillaries to the cell receptor site, bypassing the liver. This increases the likelihood of most, if not all, of the hormone being used at the cell receptor site, and little, if any, entering the liver. This reduces the likelihood of activating SHBG and liver stress.

An additional benefit is that the uptake of the hormone is far superior to the oral dosing—at least ten times better to oral dosing. Transdermal cream should be spread and rubbed in well. Care should be taken not to contaminate another person with the cream. The absolute best delivery system for transdermal is with liposome technology. Liposome technology involves wrapping the hormone with a substance called *phosphatidylcholine*, which is a naturally occurring lipid (fat) in the cell membrane. Because the cell membrane recognizes the phosphatidylcholine, the hormone passes through the cell membrane more easily.

Chapter 21: At What Age You Should Consider Bio-Identical Hormone Therapy

Generally speaking, I recommend your first assessment at least by age forty. However, I have had male patients who were suffering from low libido and erectile dysfunction, and female patients go through menopause in their mid-to-late thirties. Let me qualify this a little more. Any woman who has had a hysterectomy, has fibroids, endometriosis, or cystic breasts before the age of forty should be evaluated. Any man who suffers from low libido or erectile dysfunction prior to the age of forty should be evaluated.

There is much evidence that supporting the hormonal system with bio-identical hormones not only makes us look, feel, and function at a more youthful age than our peers, but can add many years of functional living to our lifespan. There are some well-known celebrities who benefit from natural bio-identical hormone therapy. Here are a few names you might recognize. Susanne Summers and Sylvester Stallone are both age sixty-seven, Raquel Welch is age seventy-three, and Sean Connery is age eighty-three. All of these celebrities look and function younger than their chronological age. I would say their biological ages appear approximately twenty years younger than the average American of the same age.

The great news is that you don't have to be a movie star or incredibly wealthy to take advantage of this technology. Improved skin, hair, physique, muscle mass, tone, bone density, brain function, libido, physical and sexual stamina, and more can be restored in a matter of weeks. Additionally, it is important to keep in mind that a single hormone deficiency never exists. If one hormone is deficient, or excessive, others will be as well. The hormones are intertwined like the different sections of a symphony.

Chapter 22: What Happens if I Stop Hormone Supplementation

It is important to remember that you are being supplemented with optimal physiological doses of hormones. In other words, you are being supplemented at a level of hormone that your body was capable of producing in a more youthful optimal state of health. There are specific and multiple sex hormone receptors in many different tissues: the brain, the bone, the muscles, the blood vessels, and the digestive tract, to name a few. The more receptors of a specific hormone an organ has the more dependent that particular organ is on that specific hormone. For example, the heart has more testosterone receptors than any other organ with the exception of the testes. Therefore, heart function is highly dependent upon testosterone. This is one of the reasons why heart attacks increase drastically after age fifty or so. At age fifty, the average man has lost fifty percent of the testosterone level he had at age twenty five, and, because of this alone, his risk for heart attack has doubled, independent of all other health factors.

Another example is the level of progesterone in women related to breast cancer risk. Progesterone levels start to decrease at approximately age thirty-five in women. Only five percent of breast cancer occurs in women under the age of forty. Conversely, twenty-four percent of breast cancer occurs in women who are age seventy-two and older. With each decade after age forty, the risk increases. By the time most women reach menopause (average age 51.5 years), progesterone levels are relatively low. Low progesterone levels are also related to increased osteoporosis risk in postmenopausal women as progesterone stimulates osteoblasts (new bone cell growth).

Optimum physiological dosing of bio-identical hormones helps tissues and organs to function at their best. When we stop supplementing bio-identical hormones, levels of these hormones simply return to the level that was present before supplementation was initiated. If supplementation has been used for several years, these levels may become lower than they were before supplementation began, just as they would occur in the normal aging process without supplementation. No significant adverse reactions have been documented.

After a few weeks, generally people do not feel as well as they did before when they were supplementing. The person gradually loses the added protection against inflammation, improved thinking, improved muscle tone, decreased body fat, skin and hair quality, and increased libido that they benefitted from with bio-identical supplementation. The question is do you want to look, feel, and function like an average American your age, or do you want to look, feel, and function better than your peers. Given a chance, most of us want to look and feel as good as we can for as long as we can.

When I consult with patients, they have four primary concerns about aging.

1. Will I be able to ambulate as I grow old?
2. Will I retain my mental faculties as I age?
3. Will I still appear attractive to someone (anyone) as I age?
4. Will I still be able to enjoy sex as I age?

Can bio-identical supplement help alleviate those concerns? Absolutely!

To review, there are no significant adverse risks associated with starting and later stopping bio-identical supplementation. I did so myself for about a year from age fifty-seven to fifty-eight. However, I must say, when I resumed taking the supplementation, I could see and feel a difference it made within days. Dosing with bio-identical hormones at physiological levels is safe. Transdermal dosing using liposome technology is the safest and most effective methodology available today.

Chapter 23: Symptoms/Solutions

The following is a listing of common symptoms/conditions and the possible hormone imbalances associated with them.

Signs and Symptoms	Possible Hormone Imbalances
Acne	High DHEA, testosterone
Andropause	Low GH, DHEA, High/Low cortisol, High estrogen
Anti-social behavior	Low GH
Anxiety	Low pregnenolone, progesterone, Vitamin D, melatonin; High estrogen, cortisol, thyroid
Arthritis pain	Low DHEA, cortisol, testosterone, Vitamin D, melatonin
Auto-immune disease	Low DHEA, cortisol, testosterone, Vitamin D, melatonin
Bloating, water retention	Low progesterone, High estrogen
Bone, joint, muscle pain	Low GH, DHEA, Vitamin D, High/Low cortisol
Bossiness	High DHEA, testosterone
Breast cancer	Low progesterone, Vitamin D, melatonin, High estrogen
Breast tenderness, swelling	Low progesterone, Vitamin D, High estrogen
Cancer (breast, uterus, ovarian, prostate)	Low progesterone, Vitamin D, melatonin, High estrogen
Cervical dysplasia	Low progesterone, Vitamin D, High estrogen
Chronic fatigue syndrome	Low thyroid, cortisol, testosterone, Vitamin D, melatonin
Clitoris atrophy	Low testosterone
Constipation	Low thyroid
Decreased HDL	Low progesterone, thyroid; High estrogen, testosterone

Decrease libido	Low GH, testosterone
Digestive problems	High cortisol
Dry eyes	Low DHEA
Dry skin	Low estrogen, thyroid, testosterone
Dull colors	Low pregnenelone
Endometriosis	Low progesterone; High estrogen, testosterone
Erectile Dysfunction	Low testosterone, DHEA, pregnenolone
Excessive cold (body, hands, or feet)	Low thyroid
Excessive menstrual bleeding	Low progesterone, High estrogen
Exhaustion	Low cortisol, thyroid, DHEA, testosterone, GH
Fatigue	Low cortisol, thyroid, Vitamin D, testosterone, GH
Fat, flabby muscles	Low GH, testosterone, thyroid
Fibroids	Low progesterone, High estrogen
Fibromyalgia	Low GH, testosterone, progesterone, cortisol, thyroid, Vitamin D, melatonin
Forgetfulness, fuzzy, or foggy thinking	Low pregnenolone, DHEA, testosterone, estrogen; High cortisol
Hair loss	Low thyroid, testosterone; High cortisol
Headaches	Low melatonin, thyroid; High cortisol, estrogen
Hot flashes	Low estrogen, thyroid
Hypothyroid	Low progesterone; High/Low cortisol; High estrogen
Impatience	High DHEA, testosterone
Impotence	Low GH, thyroid; High testosterone
Inability to stay awake	Low melatonin
Increased blood pressure	High cortisol, estrogen
Increased body fat	Low GH, testosterone, DHEA, thyroid;

	High cortisol, estrogen
Increased cholesterol	High cortisol, estrogen; Low thyroid
Increased insulin resistance	Low testosterone, DHEA, GH, estrogen
Inflammation	Low DHEA, cortisol, GH, testosterone; High estrogen
Insomnia	Low melatonin, progesterone; High cortisol, estrogen
Irregular menstrual cycle	Low progesterone, estrogen; High testosterone
Jet lag	Low melatonin
Lack of confidence	Low testosterone
Lack of energy	Low GH, testosterone, cortisol, thyroid, Vitamin D; High cortisol
Lightheadedness when standing after sitting or lying	Low cortisol, aldosterone
Loss of libido	(male) Low GH, testosterone, DHEA, cortisol; High estrogen; (female) Low GH, testosterone, cortisol, estrogen, progesterone
Lack of menstruation	Low estrogen
Loss of muscle	Low estrogen
Loss of nipple sensitivity	Low testosterone
Lack of orgasm	Low testosterone
Loss of self-esteem	Low testosterone
Loss of sexual interest	(female) Low GH, testosterone, estrogen, progesterone, cortisol; (male) Low GH, testosterone, DHEA, cortisol, High/Low estrogen
Low blood pressure	Low cortisol, aldosterone
Moodiness	Low DHEA, melatonin
Multiple sclerosis	Low pregnenelone, DHEA, cortisol, Vitamin D
Muscle pain	Low thyroid, Vitamin D; High cortisol

Night sweats	Low estrogen
Nervousness	Low pregnenelone, progesterone, melatonin, Vitamin D; High estrogen
Oily facial skin	High DHEA, testosterone
Osteopenia/osteoporosis	Low estrogen, progesterone, DHEA, testosterone, Vitamin D
Over confidence	High testosterone
Painful intercourse	(female) Low estrogen
Penis atrophy	Low testosterone
Poor stress management	Low DHEA, cortisol
Post traumatic stress syndrome	Low GH, pregnenolone, DHEA, testosterone, melatonin, Vitamin D, cortisol
Sagging breasts	Low estrogen
Sagging skin	Low GH, testosterone, estrogen; High cortisol
Shaking hands	High thyroid
Slow heartbeat	Low cortisol, thyroid
Stressed out	Low DHEA, High/Low cortisol
Sugar metabolism problems	High cortisol; Low testosterone, Vitamin D
Thinning hair	Low thyroid
Thinning eyebrows	(medial) Low testosterone; (middle) Low DHEA; (outer) Low thyroid
Traumatic brain injury	Low GH, pregnenolone, DHEA, testosterone, cortisol, Vitamin D, melatonin
Trembling	High thyroid
Unexplained weight loss	High thyroid
Uterine fibroids	Low progesterone, High estrogen
Urinary incontinence/infection	Low estrogen
Vaginal atrophy/dryness	Low estrogen

Waking up in the middle of the night	Low melatonin, High cortisol
Water retention	High estrogen
Water weight gain pre-menses	Low progesterone; High estrogen
Weight gain in waist, hips, thighs	Low GH, testosterone, DHEA, thyroid; High cortisol, estrogen

Chapter 24: Your Next Step

If you have read this book, you are either considering or have already made the decision to try bio-identical hormone therapy. Hopefully you have been able to understand most, if not all, of the information provided. You should feel assured that this is a safe approach to help better your health. Natural bio-identical hormone therapy is part of a functional aging approach. It is the absolute solution for a wide variety of symptoms.

I think it is important to summarize some of the key points that you have learned.

- There are three methods of testing the sex hormones—blood, urine, and saliva.
  - Saliva testing is the most accurate and least expensive.
  - Saliva testing measures the free hormones.
- Synthetic and bio-identical hormones are not the same.
  - Synthetic sex hormones have been associated with increased risk of heart attack and stroke, blood clots, and some cancers.
  - Bio-identical hormones in physiological doses are not associated with the above risks.
- There are five methods of administering the sex hormones— injections, surgically implanted pellets, oral dosing, transdermal patches, and transdermal creams.
  - Seventy percent of physicians recommend the transdermal creams.
  - Transdermal creams have at least 10 times better absorption compared to oral doses.
  - Injections, pellets, and oral dosing are more likely to cause supra-physiological hormone levels causing SHBG production from the liver.
  - Transdermal creams using liposome technology are the safest because of the first pass technology and best absorption and less likely to activate SHGB
- Hormone levels can be in reference range and still be sub-optimal.
- The hypothalamus regulates the thyroid and sex hormones through the pituitary via the H-P-T, H-P-A, or H-P-G axis.
  - The hypothalamus works similar to a thermostat by secreting or not secreting releasing hormones.

- The sex hormones are dependent upon a healthy working relationship and balance of the thyroid and adrenal glands.
  - The sex hormone levels will lower if there is low thyroid function.
  - The sex hormone levels will lower if there is prolonged cortisol production from stress.
  - Chronic cortisol production can be caused by emotional, chemical, or mechanical stress or lack of sleep.
- Type II hypothyroidism due to thyroid receptor resistance is common.
- Dried blood spot testing is more accurate than serum blood testing for the thyroid hormones.
- Hormone levels can be optimal but hypo-function can still occur in the body due to hormone receptor resistance.
  - Optimum hormone function is dependent upon optimal hormone levels coupled with optimum hormone receptor sensitivity.
- Optimum hormone function can reduce the risk for diabetes, osteoporosis, auto-immune diseases, cardiovascular disease, dementia, and certain cancers.
- The brain has receptors for all the hormones.
  - Optimum hormone function enhances memory and cognitive functions.
- Men and women have the same hormones, just the quantities are different.
- Menopause occurs when a woman ceases to have her menstrual cycle, about age fifty, on average.
- Andropause, the male version of menopause, occurs when a man has lost fifty percent of his peak testosterone levels, at about age fifty, on average.
- Somatopause occurs when an individual has lost fifty percent of their growth hormone peak levels, at about age fifty, on average.
- Genetic variances, environmental toxins, what you eat, what you drink, how you rest, how you exercise, what/how you breathe, and what you think influence your hormone function.

- Bio-identical hormone therapy can improve the quality of aging.
- Bio-identical hormone therapy is safe in physiological doses.

The first step to see if your hormones are causing your unwanted symptoms is to get a saliva hormone test to evaluate the sex hormones and dried blood spot test to evaluate the thyroid hormones and Vitamin D. These tests help to determine if you have an imbalance in your hormone system that is causing your complaints. If you want to preserve or restore your muscle mass, bone density, cognitive function, skin texture, libido, sexual performance, energy level, enthusiasm, creativity, sense of well-being, and reduce your cardiovascular risk and risk of certain cancers, then you should get started today.

For more information, to ask a question, order a test kit, or to make an appointment, visit my website at www.drkellymiller.com.

Appendix

Glossary

A

ACTH (adrenocorticotrophic hormone)—stimulating hormone produced by pituitary gland hat goes to the adrenal gland and stimulates hormone production.

Acute myocardial infarction—acute heart attack. One third of all first heart attacks are fatal.

Adaptogens—herbs that facilitate increased function of an endocrine gland like the adrenal, thyroid, or gonads.

Addison's disease—severe under-functioning of adrenal glands that can be life threatening.

ADHD (Attention Deficit Hyperactivity Disorder)—an imbalance of neurotransmitters, triggered by food/chemical/environmental allergies/sensitivities and nutritional deficiencies.

Adrenal cortex—part of the adrenal gland that produces the mineralocorticoids, such as aldosterone; the glucocorticoids like cortisol; and the sex hormones like pregnenolone, DHEA and androstenedione.

Adrenal glands—two triangular, hat-shaped glands on top of the kidneys that produce many hormones.

Adrenal medulla—center part of the adrenal gland that produces adrenaline and noradrenaline.

Adrenaline—also known as epinephrine.

Adrenimium—homeopathic preparation for the adrenal glands.

Aldosterone—mineralocorticoid responsible for body fluid balance through the regulation of sodium and potassium.

Alpha-ketoglutarate—chemical component of the mitochondrial energy cycle.

Alpha lipoic acid—anti-oxidant used in the mitochondrial energy cycle. It possesses the ability to recycle many other anti-oxidants.

A.L.S. (Amyotrophic Lateral Sclerosis a.k.a. Lou Gehrig's disease)—neurodegenerative disease of the myelin sheath, usually fatal within a few years after diagnosis.

Alzheimer's disease—neurodegenerative disease of the brain, involving the deposition of beta-amyloid plaques. It is the fastest growing cause of death in the US.

Amalgum—fillings containing silver and mercury.

Andropause—male version of menopause, occurring when there has been a fifty percent or more loss of testosterone in a man from his peak. It usually occurs around age fifty.

Androstenediol—intermediary compound involved in the conversion of DHEA to testosterone.

Androstendione—intermediary compound that can convert to estrone, testosterone, or cortisol, depending upon the physiological requirements, nutritional status, and genetic variants of the individual

Apoptosis—cell death.

Arrythmias—abnormal beating of the heart, often due to nutritional and/or hormonal deficiencies.

Arsenic—heavy metal that can be found in some water supplies, usually well water.

Aromatase—enzyme that converts testosterone to estradiol and adrostendione to estrone.

Aromatization—chemical process involving the aromatase enzyme.

Aspartame—dangerous artificial sweetener used in many diet foods.

Astralagus—herb that is an adaptogen for both the adrenals and the thyroid.

Atherogenesis—process of producing soft plaque in the arteries.

Atheromas—area of soft plaque in the arteries.

ATP (adenosine triphosphate)— cellular energy unit produced by the mitochondria from protein and carbohydrate.

Ayurvedic Medicine—traditional medicine of the Eastern Indian people that is over 2,000 years old.

B

Beta-amyloid—protein produced in the cell membrane of the neurons and other tissues.

Beta-endorphins—certain chemicals produced in the brain that have an euphoric effect.

Beta cells—specific cells in the pancreas responsible for producing insulin.

Biests—hormone formulas containing both estradiol and estriol.

Bio-circadian—the twenty-four hour biological clock in the human body.

Bio-identical—exogenous hormone that is the exact duplicate of what the body makes.

BMI (Body Mass Index)—mathematical number denoting certain health risks. It is arrived at by multiplying height and weight.

B pattern—large percentage of VLDLs in the LDL pool that increases the cardiovascular risk.

Bromine—part of the halide family in the periodic table. It can bind to iodine receptor sites and disrupt thyroid function, can be found in many plastics, in some bread, and in some soft and sport drinks.

B Vitamins—group of substances essential for the working of certain enzymes in the body. While often co-occurring in foods, each B Vitamin does something different.

C

Calcitonin—hormone produced by the thyroid that participates in calcium and phosphorus metabolism, opposes/balances parathyroid hormone functions.

Carcinogenic—substances that increase the risk of cancer cells forming.

Catecholamines—group of chemicals produced by the adrenal medulla, including dopamine, epinephrine, and norepinephrine that act as neurotransmitters and hormones.

C.B.C.—complete blood cell count, both red blood cells and white blood cells, including differentiation.

Centenarians—individuals who live to be one hundred or more years.

Chinese Traditional Medicine—traditional medicine of the Chinese people, encompassing acupuncture, spinal adjustments, and herbology. It is over two thousand years old.

Chlorine—chemical found in small amounts in the body. It is in the halide family like iodine and in excess amounts is toxic.

Cholesterol—precursor to the sex hormones and Vitamin D. It is essential to all cells in the body. Excesses and deficiencies can increase certain health risks

Chrysin—naturally occurring flavone found in certain herbs and foods.

Coenzyme Q10—nutrient essential to the mitochondrial energy cycle in every cell in the body that is inhibited by statin medications.

Cognitive loss—loss of memory and/or reasoning ability.

Congestive heart failure—condition of decreased heart cellular function, causing decreased cardiac output.

Corpus luteum—area in the ovary that produces progesterone after ovulation takes place.

Cordyceps—symbiotic relationship between a fungus and a caterpillar producing a mushroom-like structure and originally found only in Tibet.

Corticosterone—mineralocorticoid produced by the adrenal cortex from progesterone and is a precursor to aldosterone.

Cortisol—hormone produced from the adrenal cortex that has glucose forming and anti-inflammatory properties.

COMT (catechol-o-methyltransferase)—methylating enzyme that is involved in the breakdown of dopamine, epinephrine, norepinephrine, and estrogen.

COX2 (cyclooxygenase-2)—enzyme that acts to speed up the production of certain chemical messengers called prostaglandins that play a key role in in promoting inflammation.

Cross-contamination—occurs when someone using a transdermal hormone product transfers it to another person by skin contact because it was not rubbed in well and/or the other person came in contact too soon after application.

Cruciferous vegetables—vegetable family that includes broccoli, Brussels sprouts, cauliflower, and kale that aid in estrogen detoxification.

Cushing's disease—most common problem involving the adrenal cortex, associated with high blood sugars, excessive trunk weight and moon-face.

Cyanocobolamin—cheap form of B12 containing a cyanide molecule that must be methylated before it can be used in the body.

CYP1A1—enzyme involved in phase I xenobiotic and drug metabolism.

CYP1B1—enzyme involved in many reactions involved in drug metabolism and synthesis of cholesterol, steroids and other lipids

CYP450—largest family of enzymes. This superfamily of proteins contains a heme (iron) cofactor and, therefore, are hemoproteins.

D

Delta-5-pathway—enzymatic pathway involved in the conversion of cholesterol to pregnenolone.

Delta-6-pathway—enzymatic pathway involved in the conversion of these hormones.

Dementia (also known as senility)—It is a loss of cognitive function and reasoning ability.

DHEA (dehydroepiandrosterone)—hormone naturally made in the adrenal cortex. It can also be made from chemicals found in wild yam for exogenous use.

DHT (dehihydrotestosterone)—sex steroid and androgen hormone that is synthesized from testosterone in the prostate, testes, hair follicles, and adrenal glands.

DIM (diindolylmethane)—chemical formed in the body from plant substances contained in cruciferous vegetables, such as cabbage, Brussels sprouts, cauliflower, and broccoli.

Distal tubules of the kidneys—portion of kidney partly responsible for the regulation of potassium, sodium, calcium, and pH. It is also the primary site for the kidney's regulation of calcium.

Dopamine—chemical produced primarily in the frontal lobes of the brain that plays several important roles in the brain and body.

E

E4/E4—specific homozygous gene pattern that increases the risk for cardiovascular disease and Alzheimer's.

Endocrine disruptors—environmental chemicals that interfere with the body's hormone system and produce negative developmental, reproductive, neurological, and immune effects in both humans and wildlife.

Endogenous—produced by metabolic synthesis in the body.

Endometriosis—disease in which tissue that normally grows inside the uterus grows outside it.

Endometrium—mucous membrane that lines the inside of uterus.

Endoplasmic reticulum—membrane network within the cytoplasm of cells involved in the synthesis, modification, or transport of cellular materials.

Enzyme—bio-electrical molecular structure containing vitamins and minerals that transforms one chemical into another by adding or subtracting bonds.

EPF (Epidermal Growth Factor)—growth factor produced by the liver from growth hormone that stimulates cell growth, proliferation, and differentiation.

Epigenetic expression—variation of gene expression that is caused by external or environmental factors that switch genes on and off and affect how cells read genes.

Epinephrine—hormone/neurotransmitter produced by the adrenal medulla that is involved in the regulation of the sympathetic nervous system (fight/flight syndrome). It is also called adrenaline.

Erectile dysfunction— sexual dysfunction characterized by the inability to develop or maintain an erection of the penis.

Erythrocytosis—increase in the total red blood cell mass.

Esophagitis—inflammation of the esophagus, often secondary to decreased stomach secretion of HCL.

Estradiol—dominant and largest pool of estrogen in women in child-bearing years. It exists in a pool with estrone and is known as E2.

Estriol—end of the cascade of the sex hormones, the smallest fraction of estrogen, the benign form of estrogen known as E3.

Estrogen—converted from testosterone in the ovaries, the largest quantity of hormone in young females.

Estrone—hormone that exists in a pool with estradiol and is directly related to body fat, especially in men. Its metabolites are potentially carcinogenic.

Eunuchoid—resembling a eunuch, typically in having reduced sexual characteristics.

Exogenous—from an external source.

Exracellular—outside the cell.

Extraterrestial—not part of normal biological systems.

F

4-nonylphenol—used in a variety of pesticides and consumer products and a common biodegradation product of detergents. 4-Nonylphenol mimics estrogen and is, therefore, an endocrine-disrupting compound.

Fibroids—non-cancerous (benign) tumors that grow from the muscle layers of the uterus.

First pass—refers to the fact that the sublingual or transdermal nutraceutical/hormone is taken directly to the receptor sites in the cells without going through digestion and the liver.

Fluoride—common ingredient in mouthwash and toothpaste that competes for iodine receptor sites and is accumulative and toxic.

Foam cells—macrophage (specific type of white blood cell) that has absorbed fat and cholesterol in the blood vessel.

Fosamax—prescription medication for osteoporosis that has a half-life of ten years and has been associated with esophagitis and spontaneous fractures of the hip.

FSH (follicular stimulating hormone)—stimulating hormone produced from the pituitary that causes ovulation.

G

GABA (gamma-aminobutyric acid)—neurotransmitter in the brain. Fifty percent of the world's population is GABA-dominant.

GDP-choline—nutraceutical that increases growth hormone production.

Glucocorticoids—hormones produced by the adrenal cortex that causes increased glucose production.

Glucose—name for the type of sugar the body uses to convert into ATP in the mitochondria.

Glycemic—measurement of glucose in foods and its effect on physiology and bio-chemistry.

Goiter—nodular mass in the thyroid usually due to iodine deficiency.

Gonadotrophic releasing hormone—hormone released from the hypothalamus that causes the pituitary to release leutinizing and follicular stimulating hormones to the testes/ovaries.

Gonads—testicles or ovaries.

Growth hormone—master hormone known as the "battery" hormone that has influence over growth and the other hormones and neurotransmitters.

GST (glutathione-s-transferase)—enzyme with common gene variants that is used in estrogen detoxification.

Gymnema—herb used in Ayurvedic Medicine for hundreds of years that stimulates new pancreatic beta cell production.

Halcion—prescription anti-depressant.

Half-life—length of time it takes fifty percent of a drug to be metabolized.

Halides—group of elements in the periodic table that share certain properties. Iodine, chlorine, bromine, and fluoride represent the halides.

Hashimoto's disease (thyroiditis)—causes hypothyroidism due to autoimmune disease from the TPO antibody.

HDL (high density lipoproteins)—the larger carrier lipoproteins for cholesterol, known as "good" cholesterol. There are five different kinds of HDLs.

HFCS (high fructose corn syrup)—common food additive of fructose derived from corn sugar. It is a neurotoxin that must be broken down in the liver.

Homeopathic—diluted amount of a substance that can be toxic at high levels but helps heal at minute dosages. Homeopathy is a three hundred year old health care discipline known to work by "the law of similar".

Homocysteine—by-product of the amino acid, methione, metabolism. It is an inflammatory marker for cardiovascular disease.

H-P-A axis—hypothalamus, pituitary, and adrenal hormone interactions.

H-P-G axis—hypothalamus, pituitary, and gonadal hormone interactions.

H-P-T axis—hypothalamus, pituitary, and thyroid hormone interactions.

Hydrochlorhydria—decreased ability to secrete hydrochloric acid in the stomach.

Hydroxylation—process of adding a hydroxyl ion (OH-) to a molecule to make it more water soluble for the purpose of detoxification.

Hyperinsulinism—excess insulin production in response to blood glucose levels.

Hypogonadism—clinical diagnosis of hormone production from the testes or ovaries that is below reference ranges.

Hypothalamus—endocrine organ in the brain that monitors internal sensory data from the gonads, thyroid, and adrenals.

Hypothyroidism—decreased function of the thyroid, a common condition often undiagnosed by health care providers.

I

I-3-C (indole-3–carbinol)—substance found in broccoli, Brussels sprouts, cauliflower, kale, cabbage, mustards greens, collard greens, turnips, and rutabagas that is important in estrogen detoxification.

IGF-1 (Insulin Growth Factor I)—hormone produced by the liver from growth hormone that is similar in molecular structure to insulin. It plays an important role in childhood growth and continues to have anabolic effects in adults.

IGF-2 (Insulin Growth Factor II)—one of three protein hormones that share structural similarity to insulin, produced from growth hormone in the liver.

IL-1—group of 11 cytokines that plays a central role in the regulation of immune and inflammatory responses to infections or sterile insults.

IL-6—interleukin that has both pro-inflammatory and anti-inflammatory properties. In humans, it is encoded by the *IL6* gene.

iNOS—inducible nitric oxide synthase, both tumoricidal and bactericidal, mediates COX2.

Insulin resistance—generally regarded as a pathological condition in which cells fail to respond to the normal actions of the hormone insulin.

Inverse correlation—contrary relationship between two variables such that they move in opposite directions.

Iodide—salt of hydriotic acid consisting of two elements, one of which is iodine, as sodium iodide.

Iodine—a halide in the elemental chart and an essential micronutrient for the body. It is in high concentrations in the thyroid, breasts, uterus, and prostate.

L

LDL (low density lipoproteins)—the smaller carrier for cholesterol, known as the "bad" cholesterol. There are seven different kinds of LDLs.

Leaky gut (also known as hyperpermeability)—phenomenon whereby the intestine wall exhibits permeability. This condition causes many food/chemical allergies/sensitivities and autoimmune disease.

Leptin (the "satiety hormone")—hormone made by adipose cells that helps to regulate energy balance by inhibiting hunger. Leptin is opposed by the actions of the hormone ghrelin, the "hunger hormone".

Levothyroxine—prescription medicine of the synthetic form of T4.

Leydig cells (interstitial cells of Leydig)—found adjacent to the seminiferous tubules in the testicle. They produce testosterone when stimulated by luteinizing hormone (LH).

LH (luteinizing hormone)—hormone produced by the pituitary that stimulates testosterone in men and estrogen in women.

Licorice Root (root of *Glycyrrhiza glabra*)—an adaptogen that supports adrenal function. It should be used with caution in individuals with high blood pressure.

Lipitor—brand name for a prescription statin medication.

Lipoprotein A (a type of LDL)—increased risk factor for atherosclerotic diseases, such as coronary heart disease and stroke.

Liposome—technology of enveloping a nutrient or hormone with phosphotidylcholine.

Lipotropin—hormone produced by the anterior pituitary gland that promotes the breakdown of lipids stored in the body's fat cells.

Lisinopril—drug known as an angiotensin-converting enzyme (ACE) inhibitor used in treatment of high blood pressure and heart failure.

M

Melanocyte-stimulating hormone—derived from a protein known as proopiomelanocortin (POMC) and secreted primarily by the pituitary gland.

Mercury—chemical element with symbol Hg. Mercury poisoning can result from exposure to water-soluble forms of mercury (mercuric chloride or methylmercury), by inhalation of mercury vapor, amalgam fillings, or by eating large ocean fish and high fructose corn syrup contaminated with mercury.

Metabolic syndrome—group of risk factors that include high blood pressure, high blood sugar, unhealthy cholesterol levels, and abdominal fat. It is estimated 47 million Americans have it.

Metabolites—substances produced by metabolism or by a metabolic process.

Methylation—process in which 'methyl groups' (CH3) are added to a compound in the body. It is a necessary process in estrogen detoxification and many essential body functions. It is a common deficiency in America due to genetic variants, nutritional deficiencies, and excess body burden of environmental toxins.

Methylcobolamin—better form of Vitamin B12. It differs from cyanocobalamin in that the cyanide is replaced with a methyl group.

Methylmalonic acid—compound that reacts with Vitamin B12 to produce coenzyme A (CoA). Coenzyme A is essential to normal mitochondrial cellular function.

Melatonin—substance found in all animals, plants, fungi, and bacteria. It is the oldest hormone on the planet. The hormone can be used as a sleep aid and in the treatment of some sleep disorders. It is the most powerful anti-oxidant in the body.

Mineralocorticoids—corticoid steroid like aldosterone that is produced in the adrenal cortex and manages fluid balances in the body by changing sodium/potassium balance.

Mitochondria—organelles found in large numbers in most cells, the "power plant" of the cell. There are thousands in a cell, the numbers controlled by the thyroid gland.

MMPS—calcium-dependent zinc-containing enzymes. Collectively, these enzymes are capable of degrading all kinds of extracellular matrix proteins, but also can process a number of bioactive molecules. MMPs are also thought to play a major role in cell behaviors, such as cell proliferation migration (adhesion/dispersion), differentiation, angiogenesis, apoptosis, and host defense.

Morphine—pain medication of the opiate type. It acts directly on the central nervous system (CNS) to decrease the feeling of pain. It is highly addictive.

MRT (Mediator Release Test)—blood analysis to determine food/chemical allergy/sensitivity.

MSG (monosodium glutamate)—used in the food industry and Asian foods as a flavor enhancer that has an umami taste to intensify the meaty, savory flavor of food, as a naturally occurring glutamate does in foods such as stews and meat soups. It is an excitotoxin and is particularly dangerous to the fetus and children.

MTHFR—gene that provides instructions for making an enzyme called methylenetetrahydrofolate reductase. This enzyme plays a role in processing amino acids, the building blocks of proteins. It is a common gene variant in the population.

Myopathy—muscular disease in which the muscle fibers do not function for any one of many reasons, resulting in muscular weakness.

N

Nanotechnology—manipulation of matter on an atomic, molecular, and supramolecular scale to make it smaller and more easily absorbed.

Natural killer cells—cells that can react against and destroy another cell without prior sensitization to it. NK cells are part of our first line of defense against cancer cells and virus-infected cells.

Negative feedback—some function of the output of a system, process, or mechanism is fed back in a manner that tends to reduce the fluctuations in the output, whether caused by changes in the input or by other disturbances. This is how much of the hormone system works.

Nettles—herb used for centuries to treat allergy symptoms, particularly hayfever, which is the most common allergy problem. It contains biologically active compounds that reduce inflammation and inhibit the aromatase enzyme reducing the conversion of testosterone to estrogen.

NGF (Neural Growth Factor)—made by the liver from growth hormone. It is primarily involved in the regulation of growth, maintenance, proliferation, and survival of certain target neurons.

Neuropathy—damage to or disease affecting nerves, which may impair sensation, movement, gland or organ function, or other aspects of health, depending on the type of nerve affected. Common causes include systemic diseases (such as diabetes or leprosy), vitamin deficiency, medication (such as chemotherapy), traumatic injury, radiation therapy, excessive alcohol consumption, immune system disease, Celiac disease, or viral infection.

Neurotransmitters (chemical messengers in the brain)—endogenous chemicals that enable neurotransmission. They trasmit signals across a chemical synapse, such as a neuromuscular junction, from one nerve cell to another "target" nerve cell, muscle cell, or gland cell.

NIDDM (Non-insulin dependent diabetic)—former name for type 2 diabetes mellitus.

Nitric oxide—important cellular signaling molecule involved in many physiological and pathological processes. It is a powerful vasodilator with a short half-life of a few seconds in the blood and is essential to normal endothelial (vascular cell) function.

Nor-adrenaline—catecholamine that is a neurotransmitter and also a neuro-hormone produced by the adrenal medulla in response to sympathetic nervous system stimulation, primarily in response to hypotension. It produces an increase in heart rate and elevation of blood pressure.

Norepinephrine—another name for noradrenaline.

O

Opioid—chemical similar to the alkaloid found in opium poppies. Historically they have been used as painkillers and are highly addictive. They stimulate dopamine, the 'feel good' neurotransmitter in the frontal brain.

Ornithine—non-essential amino acid derived from the breakdown of arginine during the mitochondrial energy cycle. It helps build muscle and reduce body fat, especially when combined with the amino acids arginine and carnitine. Ornithine is also needed for the formation of citrulline, proline, and glutamic acid—three amino acids that help supply energy to every cell in the body.

Osteoblasts—cell arising from a fibroblast and is associated with bone production.

Osteopenia – a condition in which bone mineral density is lower than normal. It is a precursor to osteoporosis.

Osteoporosis—decreased bone strength tht increases the risk of a broken bone. It is the most common reason for a broken bone among the elderly.

P

PBAs—chemical used in many plastic products, including bottle water, soda, and storage containers for food leftovers. This harmful chemical can adversely affect the endocrine, nervous, and immune systems.

PCBs—synthetic, organic chlorine compound derived from biphenyl. Polychlorinated biphenyls were widely used in electrical apparatus, cutting fluids for machining operations, carbonless copy paper, and in heat transfer fluids. Because of PCBs environmental toxicity and classification as a persistent organic pollutant, the U.S. Congress banned PCB production in 1979, and the Stockholm Convention on Persistent Organic Pollutants did the same in 2001. Studies show almost everyone has PCBs in their bodies.

Peperine extract—chemical responsible for the pungency of black pepper and long pepper. It increases the absorption of some nutrients.

Perimenopause—period of time before menopause and a time when the ovaries gradually begin to make less estrogen. It usually starts in a woman's 40s, but can start in her 30s or even earlier.

Peuraria Mirifica—herb plant that has been used in Thailand for medicinal purposes for many years, mainly as a female hormone supplement. Pueraria mirifica contains a compound called miroestrol. It helps hot flashes, vaginal dryness, and sleep in peri- and menopausal women.

Phenotype—set of observable characteristics of an individual resulting from the interaction of its genotype with the environment.

Phosphatidylcholine—integral component of the cell membrane in every cell in the human body. Phosphatidylcholine has been shown to play a vital role in many important areas including maintaining cell structure, fat metabolism, memory, nerve signalling and as a precursor to important neurotransmitters and liver health. It is part of liposome technology.

Physiological dosing—dosing with bio-identical hormones at a level that the body could naturally produce in a younger, optimal state.

Pituitary—tiny organ, the size of a pea, found at the base of the brain. As the "master gland" of the body, it produces many hormones that stimulate the thyroid, adrenal, and gonads to produce other hormones.

PMOC (proopiomelanocortin)—cleaved to give rise to multiple peptide hormones.

Polymorphism—existing in several different forms.

Positive feedback—process in which a change from the normal range elicits a response that amplifies or enhances that change. This is how a woman's production of estrogen and progesterone are controlled.

Postural hypotension—drop in blood pressure (hypotension) due to a change in body position (posture) when a person moves from sitting to standing or from lying down to sitting or standing. It is an indicator of adrenal fatigue.

Precursor—molecular structure that comes before another structure of a similar kind that is changed by an enzymatic reaction.

Pregnenolone—first sex hormone converted from cholesterol in the mitochondria of the adrenal cortex.

Pregnenolone steal—term denoting that the majority of conversion of pregnenolone is occurring through progesterone to cortisol due to a stress reaction and, subsequently, the pathway to DHEA and testosterone is inhibited causing decreased production of these two anabolic hormones.

Progesterone—sex hormone converted from pregnenoline that balances estrogen in women and converts to testosterone in men.

Progestin—synthetic prescription form of progesterone that has markedly less efficient binding capabilities and has been associated with increased cardiovascular and estrogen-related cancer risks.

Protomorphogen—dehydrated glandular extract usually from a sheep or bovine source that helps in healing and repair of that specific organ.

PSA (prostate –specific antigen)—protein produced by prostate cells. The PSA test is done to help diagnose and follow prostate cancer in men.

Q

Quercetin—bioflavonoid common in the plant kingdom, especially high in onions, red wine, and green tea. Quercetin acts as a potent polyphenol antioxidant and immune system modulator. Many of its immune support attributes are enhanced by its synergistic relationship with Vitamin C. It is highly active in the skin and lining of the digestive tract.

R

Ragland's test—simple test that can be done to see if a person has a possible problem with adrenal glands. This is the procedure. Lie on your back for 3-5 minutes then have your blood pressure taken. Stand up and immediately have your blood pressure taken again. If the systolic (the first number) doesn't rise at least 4 to 10 points, hypoadrenia is suspected. If your pressure drops, it is confirmatory for adrenal fatigue.

Receptor resistance—decreased efficiency of a hormone binding to the receptor site on the cell membrane.

Relative androgen deficiency—deficiency of DHEA and/or testosterone as evidenced by loss of function even though levels may be within a laboratory reference range.

Releasing hormone—hormone produced and secreted by the hypothalamus that signals the pituitary to secrete the corresponding stimulating hormone.

Resveratrol—type of natural phenol, produced naturally by several plants with anti-oxidant properties. Food sources of resveratrol include the skin of grapes, blueberries, raspberries, and mulberries.

Rickets—defective mineralization or calcification of bones before epiphyseal closure due to deficiency or impaired metabolism of Vitamin D, phosphorus or calcium, potentially leading to fractures and deformity. Rickets is among the most frequent childhood diseases in many developing countries and is increasing in the US.

rT3 (Reverse triiodothyronine or 3, 3', 5'-triiodothyronine, reverse T_3, or rT_3)—isomer of triiodothyronine (3,5, 3' triiodothyronine, T_3). It occurs naturally to get rid of excess T4 in the body. Problems arise when the normal 10-20% production increases to 50% or more as it is not bio-active to the cell receptor. Too much rT3 will cause a hypothyroid function despite having TSH and total T3 levels within reference range.

S

Scurvy—condition caused by a lack of Vitamin C in the diet. Signs of scurvy include tiredness, muscle weakness, joint and muscle aches, a rash on the legs, and bleeding gums.

Selenium—trace mineral necessary to all functions of the body. This important nutrient is vital to immune system function. It works in conjunction with Vitamin E, Vitamin C, glutathione, and Vitamin B3 as an antioxidant to prevent free radical damage in the body and along with zinc is necessary for the conversion of T4 to T3.

Secretagogues—substance that causes a gland to secrete another substance.

Secretory IgA—principal agent of mucosal immunity that lines the digestive tract. Decreased amounts are caused by prolonged excess cortisol production and decreased DHEA levels.

Serotonin—one of the main neurotransmitters in the brain that is responsible for feeling calm and sense of well-being. Seventeen percent of the world's population is serotonin dominant.

Sex hormones – hormones such as estrogen and testosterone that affect the growth or function of the reproductive organs, the development of secondary sex characteristics, and the reproductive behavior.

SHGB (sex hormone binding globulin)—protein that binds to and transports sex hormones like testosterone and estrogen through the bloodstream. When SHBG is bound to testosterone or estrogen, these hormones cannot stimulate cell recptors.

Stimulating hormone—hormone produced and secreted by the pituitary gland that signals the adrenals, thyroid, or gonads to produce a particular hormone.

SNP (Single nucleotide polymorphism)—genetic polymorphism between two genomes that is based on deletion, insertion, or exchange of a single nucleotide. It is the most common form of genetic variance.

Somatopause—gradual and progressive decrease in growth hormone secretion that occurs normally with increasing age during adult life and is associated with an increase in adipose tissue and LDL levels and a decrease in lean body mass.

Spermatozoa—motile sperm cell.

St. John's Wort—medicinal herb with antidepressant activity and potent anti-inflammatory properties.

Sub-lingual—under the tongue dosing directly into the bloodstream.

Supra-physiological—higher level than the body is capable of naturally producing.

Syndrome X—group of risk factors including high blood pressure, high blood sugar, high triglycerides, low HDL cholesterol, and belly fat that increases risk of heart disease and diabetes.

Synthetic hormone—extraterrestrial molecule that has been developed by a pharmaceutical company to mimic a natural hormone, but has side effects when used.

Synthroid—prescription synthetic form of T4.

TD (tardive dyskinesia)—mostly irreversible neurological disorder of involuntary movements caused by long-term use of antipsychotic or neuroleptic drugs.

Tight junctions—lateral cell membranes of adjacent cells, limiting trans-epithelial permeability in the small intestine and limiting trans-endothelial permeability in the blood-brain barrier.

T3 – triiodothyronine—bioactive form of thyroid hormone that is converted from T4 in the liver.

T4-thyroxine—one of the primary the hormones produced by the thyroid gland that is highly dependent upon adequate iodine.

Target organ—organ, such as thyroid, adrenals or gonads that receives the stimulating hormone from the pituitary or the organ that produces the hormones after stimulation.

Testosterone—predominant hormone in younger men. It is converted from DHEA or progesterone through intermediaries.

TBG (thyroid binding globulin)—globulin that binds thyroid hormones in circulation. It is one of three proteins along with transthyretin and serum albumin responsible for carrying the thyroid hormones thyroxine (T_4) and 3,5,3'-triiodothyronine (T_3) in the bloodstream. Once bound, the T4 and T3 are not bio-available to stimulate the cell receptors.

Thyroid—one of the largest endocrine glands that consists of two connected lobes. It is found in the anterior neck below the Adam's apple. The thyroid gland controls the metabolic and the body's sensitivity to other hormones.

Thyroiditis—inflammation of the thyroid gland.

Thyroxine—thyroid hormone that contains iodine and is a derivative of the amino acid tyrosine. It is formed and stored in the thyroid follicles as thyroglobulin and released from the gland by the action of an enzyme. It is converted to triiodothyronine (T3) in the liver and has a greater biological activity than T4.

Trans-fats—type of unsaturated fats that are uncommon in nature but became commonly produced industrially from vegetable fats for use in margarine, snack food, packaged baked goods and frying fast food. Trans-fat has been shown to consistently be associated, in an intake-dependent way, with increased risk of coronary heart disease by disrupting normal cell membrane functions producing inflammation.

TGF (Transfer Growth Factor)—one of six growth factors produced in the liver from growth hormone.

TNFa—produced primarily by cells of the immune system, capable of causing hemorrhagic necrosis of certain tumor cells but not normal cells. They also destroy cells associated with the inflammatory response.

Triclosan—an antibacterial and antifungal agent found in consumer products, including toothpaste, soaps, detergents, toys, and surgical cleaning treatments. It is an endocrine disruptor.

Triests—synthetic hormones used in the past containing estrone, estradiol, and estriol that increases the risk of cardiovascular complications and breast cancer.

TPO (thyroid peroxidase)—enzyme involved in thyroid hormone synthesis. Elevated levels indicate an autoimmune response.

Transdermal—the application of a hormone or nutrient through the skin so that it is absorbed better into the body.

Tryptophan—amino acid that is found in many foods, such as turkey.

TSH (thyroid stimulating hormone)—most common monitor of thyroid function on routine lab tests. TSH is produced by the pituitary and has reference ranges of one thousand percent, which are much too broad.

T-score—bone density compared to the average 30-year-old man or woman.

Type II hypothyroidism—functional state of hypothyroidism despite the presence of normal reference range values for thyroid function due to a lack of cell receptor sensitivity.

Tyrosine—non-essential amino acid that helps regulate mood and stimulates the nervous system. It is necessary for optimal adrenal and thyroid function.

U

Uterus—hollow muscular organ of the female reproductive system that is responsible for the development of the embryo and fetus during pregnancy. Fibroids of the uterus become common in the aging process due to lack of progesterone.

V

Valium—medication that typically produces a calming effect. It is commonly used to treat a range of conditions, including anxiety, alcohol withdrawal syndrome, benzodiazepine withdrawal syndrome, muscle spasms, seizures, trouble sleeping, and restless leg syndrome.

VGF (Vascular Growth Factor)—substance made by the liver from growth hormone that stimulates new blood vessel formation.

Vitamin C—water-soluble vitamin needed for normal growth and development. It is needed for growth and repairs of tissues in all parts of the body. It is one of many antioxidants that block some of the damage cause by free radicals.

Vitamin D—found in small amounts in a few foods, including fatty fish such as herring, mackerel, sardines and tuna. To make Vitamin D more available, it is added to dairy products, juices, and cereals that are then said to be "fortified with Vitamin D." But most Vitamin D – 80% to 90% of what the body gets – is obtained through exposure to sunlight. Vitamin D is best absorbed in conjunction with Vitamin K2. The vast majority of Americans are deficient.

Vitamin E—found naturally in some foods and important as an anti-oxidant in the cell membrane, which is mostly fat. Natural occurring Vitamin E exists in eight forms (alpha-, beta-, gamma-, and delta-tocopherols are examples).

VLDL (very low density lipoprotein)—very small type of lipoprotein that carries cholesterol and is associated with increased cardiovascular risk. It is made by the liver.

X

Xenoestrogens—substance that imitates estrogen. They can be either synthetic or natural chemical compounds. Synthetic xenoestrogens are widely used industrial compounds, such as PCBs, BPA and phthalates, which have estrogenic effects on a living organism causing estrogen dominant health risks of increased cardiovascular risk and breast, uterine, ovarian, and prostate cancers.

Z

Zinc—essential trace mineral involved in over three hundred enzyme reactions in the body. Many individuals have a zinc deficiency.

Zona fasciculate—layer of cells in the cortical portion of the adrenal gland, between the zona glomerulosa and zona reticularis, which secretes cortisol and DHEA.

Zona glomerulosa—most superficial layer of the adrenal cortex. Cells of the zona glomerulosa produce and secrete mineralocortisoid and aldosterone into the blood to regulate blood pressure.

Zona reticularis—innermost layer of the adrenal cortex. Cells in the zona reticularis produce androgens, including DHEA and androstenedione, from cholesterol.

Z-score—comparison of a person's bone density with that of an average person of the same age and sex.

Index

A

ACTH – adrenocorticotrophic hormone, pages 38, 47, 104-105
Acute myocardial infarctions, page 136
Adaptogens, page 106
Addison's disease, page 106
ADHD, pages 67, 68
Adrenal cortex, pages 9, 10, 23-24, 37, 43, 45, 47, 49, 103-106, 140
Adrenal glands, pages 1, 4-6, 9, 10, 12-13, 23, 30-31, 34, 37-39, 42-45, 47-48, 59, 66, 68-69, 76, 80, 88-90, 103-107, 112, 114-118, 136, 140
Adrenal medulla, pages 103, 105
Adrenaline, pages 2, 66, 103, 105
Adrenimium, page 107
Aldosterone, pages 4, 9, 23, 27, 29, 37, 47-48, 103-106, 114, 159
Alpha-ketogluterate, page 98
Alpha lipoic acid, pages 68, 80
A.L.S. – Amyotrophic Lateral Sclerosis a.k.a. Lou Geghrig's disease, page 19
Alzheimer's disease, pages vii, 60, 64, 66, 127, 134
Amalgam, page 111
Andropause, pages 59, 97, 157, 164
Androstenediol, page 10
Androstendione, page 67
Apoptosis, page 121, 136
Arrhythmias, page 136
Arsenic, page 111
Aromatase, page 43, 61, 63-64, 67-68, 76, 78-80, 117
Aromatization, page 61, 78-80
Aspartame, page 1
Astragalus, page 107
Atherogenesis, page 80
Atheromas, page 80
ATP – adenosine triphosphate, page 109
Ayurvedic Medicine, page 80

B

Beta-amyloid, page 66
Beta endorphins, page 104

Beta cells, pages 67, 136
Biest, page 82
Bio-circadian, pages 125-126
Bio-identical, pages iv, vii, ix, 1-3, 12, 30, 32, 39, 60-61, 63, 77, 82, 87-88, 107, 140, 141, 149, 153, 155-156, 163, 165
B.M.I., body mass index, pages 80, 82
B pattern, pages 65, 67
B Vitamins, pages 2, 11, 17, 86, 88-90, 105-106, 113, 115-116, 118, 139
Bromine, page 111

C

Calcitonin, page 114
Carcinogenic, pages 76, 82-83, 86-87, 89
Catecholamines, page 103
C.B.C., page 65
Centenarians, pages 2, 122
Chinese Traditional Medicine, page 81
Chlorine, page 111
Cholesterol, pages vii, 3, 9, 19-21, 23, 40, 49, 66-67, 69, 76-77, 81, 96, 106-107, 112, 115, 118, 133, 135, 159
Chrysin, pages 65, 84, 89, 139
Coenzyme Q10, CoQ10, pages 80, 93
Cognitive loss, pages 19, 39, 49, 61, 96, 97, 123, 164-165
Congestive heart failure, pages 19, 30
Corpus luteum, page 75
Cordyceps, page 115
Corticosterone, page 27
Cortisol, pages 1, 3, 5, 8-12, 23-24, 27, 29, 31-33, 35, 37, 38-41, 43-45, 47, 50, 66-69, 88-90, 103-107, 114, 116-117, 121, 126, 138-140, 145-146, 157-161, 164
COMT, page 86
COX2, page 79
Cross-contamination, pages 116, 118
Cruciferous vegetables, page 86
Cushing's disease, pages 39, 106
Cyanocobalamin, page 149
CYP1A1, pages 85-86
CYP1B1, pages 85-86
CYP450, page 85

D

E

F

Fibroids, pages 28, 30-32, 35, 82, 90, 140, 153, 158, 160
First pass, pages 51, 64, 163
Fluoride, page 111
Foam cells, page 81
Fosamax, page 32
FSH – follicular stimulating hormone, pages 55-56, 64-65, 80

G

GABA, pages 68, 77-78
GDP-choline, pages 98-99
Glucocorticoids, pages 18-19, 23, 17, 37, 39, 103, 105
Glucose, pages 35, 38, 56, 65-66, 68, 104, 136
Glycemic, pages 97-98, 137
Goiter, pages 110, 115, 133
Gonadotrophic releasing hormone, pages 56
Gonads, pages 1, 5-6, 10, 105
Grave's Disease, page 113
Growth Hormone (GH), pages 3, 95-96. 99, 121, 147, 164, 157-161
GST – glutathione-s-transferase, pages 86-87
Gymnema, page 68

H

Halcion, page 124
Half-life, pages 31, 95
Halides, page 111
Hashimoto's disease, page 113
HDL – high density lipoprotein, pages 35, 66-68, 70, 76-77, 79, 136, 157
HFCS – high fructose corn syrup, page 1
Homeopathic, pages 107, 114
Homocysteine, pages 65, 68, 77, 86
H-P-A axis, pages 37, 104, 115, 118, 163
H-P-G axis, pages 75, 118, 163
H-P-T axis, pages 108, 115, 118, 163
Hyprochlorhydria, page 150
Hydroxylation, page 83
Hyperinsulinism, page 79
Hypogonadism, pages 58-59
Hypothalamus, pages 1, 5-6, 28, 38, 55-56, 59, 63, 74, 78, 95, 103-104, 108, 123, 163

Hypothyroidism, pages 6, 32-33, 90, 110-115, 164

I

I-3-C – indole-3–carbinol, pages 84-86, 88-90
IGF-1- Insulin Growth Factor-1, pages 95-97, 99
IGF-2 – Insulin Growth Factor-II, pages 95, 98
IL-1, page 135
IL-6, page 78
iNOS, page 78
Insulin resistance, pages 1,5-6, 60, 66, 79-80, 90, 136-137, 159
Inverse correlation, page 135
Iodide, page 115
Iodine, pages 110-113, 115, 153

L

Leaky gut, pages 44, 138
LDL – low density lipoprotein, pages 66-67, 69, 77-79, 81
Leptin, pages 1, 97
Levothyroxine, pages 32, 116, 118
Leydig cells, page 78
LH – luteinizing hormone, pages 55-56, 64-65, 80
Libido, pages vi, 19, 28, 31, 49, 51, 56-57, 59-60, 63, 66, 70, 78-79, 88-90, 96-97, 99, 116, 145, 153, 156-157, 159, 165
Licorice root, page 107
Lipitor, page 115
Lipoprotein A, pages 77-78
Liposome, pages 14, 16-17, 24-25, 44, 50, 64, 68, 87, 98, 137, 139, 151, 156, 163
Lipotropin, page 104-105
Lisinopril, page 115

M

Melanocyte-stimulating hormone, pages 104-105
Mercury, pages 1,12,111
Metabolic syndrome, pages 60, 65, 79, 136
Metabolites, pages 65, 76, 83-84, 86, 89, 139, 145, 147
Methylation, pages 44, 68, 83-84, 86, 88-89, 139
Methylcobalamin, page 149
Methylmalonic acid, page 86
Melatonin, pages 2, 3, 77, 121-126, 133, 157-161
Mineralocorticoids, pages 8, 18, 22, 27, 104-105

Positive feedback, pages 27, 75, 77
Postural hypotension, pages 104, 106
Precursor, pages 105, 146, 196
Pregnenolone, pages 3, 8-9, 11-12, 19-20, 23-25, 27, 31, 38, 43-44, 49-50, 65-66, 68-69, 88-89, 146, 157-160
Pregnenolone steal, pages 11, 38, 44, 50
Progesterone, pages vii, 1, 3, 8-9, 11-12, 17, 20, 22, 27-32, 34-35, 37, 39, 47, 55, 69, 75-77, 82, 88-89, 116, 118, 137, 139-140, 143-146, 155, 157-161
Progestin, page 30
Protomorphogen, pages 107, 112, 114
PSA, page 60

Q

Quercetin, page 65

R

Ragland's test, page 106
Receptor resistance, pages 1, 80
Relative androgen deficiency, page 60
Releasing hormone, pages 4-5, 38, 108
Resveratrol, pages 86, 139
Rickets, page 138
rT3, page 113

S

Scurvy, page 133
Selenium, pages 2, 110, 113-114
Secretagogues, page 96
Secretory IgA, page 44
Serotonin, pages 44, 68, 77-78, 121
Sex hormones, pages vi, vii, 3, 6, 8, 15, 18, 22, 37, 39, 43, 46, 51, 62-63, 65-66, 69, 76, 80, 89, 103, 105, 115, 121, 138, 141, 146-149, 155, 163-165
SHBG– sex hormone binding globulin, pages 15, 51, 57, 61, 63-65, 80, 149-151, 163
Stimulating hormone, page 4
SNP – single nucleotide polymorphism, page 84
Somatopause, pages 95-97, 164
Spermatozoa, page 59

St. John's Wort, page 124
Sublingual, pages 34, 44, 68, 87-89, 93, 115-116, 137, 139, 150
Supra-physiological, pages 15, 63, 149-150, 163
Syndrome X, pages 65-66, 77-80, 136-137
Synthetic hormone, pages vii, 62, 82, 149
Synthroid, page 114

T

TD –tardive dyskinesia, page 121
Tight junctions, page 44
T3 – triiodothyronine, pages 6, 34, 112-116, 118, 201
T4 – thyroxine, pages 6, 34, 112-116, 118, 201
Target organ, page 4
Testosterone, pages iv, vii, 1, 3, 5, 8, 10-13, 17-18, 20, 22, 27, 29-30, 34, 38, 43-44, 49-50, 55-57, 59-70, 76-81, 88-89, 105, 116-118, 138-140, 145, 147-150, 155, 157-161, 164
Thyroid, pages iv, 1-3, 5-6, 8, 29-30, 32, 38, 43, 55, 66, 68-69, 88-90, 95, 105, 1-9-119, 146-147, 157-161, 163-165
Thyroiditis, page 118
Thyroxine, page 6
Trans-fats, pages 1, 22, 201
TGF – Transfer Growth Factor, pages 95,98
TNFa, pages 135-136
Triclosan, page 111
Triests, page 82
TPO – thyroid peroxidase, page 82, 112-113
TRA, pages 112-113
Transdermal, pages 16-17, 24, 28-29, 31, 33, 44, 50, 58, 63-64, 68, 88-89, 118, 125, 139-140, 149-151-163
Tryptophan, page 124
TSH – thyroid stimulating hormone, pages 5, 30, 89, 111-115
T-score, page 141
Type II hypothyroidism, pages 6, 30, 113, 164
Tyrosine, pages 105-106

U

Uterus, pages 27=28, 31, 34=35, 65, 75-76, 78, 89, 110, 139-140, 145, 157

V

I found this article while doing research on the book called *Saving Our Brains: Causes, Prevention and Treatment of Dementia and Alzheimer's Disease* (pending publication) that I co-authored with one of my great mentors, Dr. Paul Ling Tai. I find it very relative to the need for micronutrient testing. Please note this article is from 1936.

"Modern Miracle Men" – Relating To Proper Food Mineral Balances by Dr. Charles Northen, Reprinted From Cosmopolitan, June 1936

Presented by Mr. Fletcher June 1 1936 and Ordered to be Printed by the United States Government Printing Office Washington: 1936 During the 74th Congress, Second Session, Document No. 264

This is the Unabridged Version of this document.

MODERN MIRACLE MEN

Dr. Charles Northen, Who Builds Health From The Ground Up

This quiet, unballyhooed pioneer and genius in the field of nutrition demonstrates that countless human ills stem from the fact that impoverished soil of America no longer provides plant foods with the mineral elements essential to human nourishment and health! To overcome this alarming condition, he doctors sick soils and, by seeming miracles, raises truly healthy and health-giving fruits and vegetables.

(By Rex Beach)

Do you know that most of us today are suffering from certain dangerous diet deficiencies which cannot be remedied until the depleted soils from which our foods come are brought into proper mineral balance?

The alarming fact is that foods — fruit and vegetables and grains — now being raised on millions of acres of land no longer contain enough of certain needed minerals, are starving us — no matter how much of them we eat!

This talk about minerals is novel and quite startling. In fact, a realization of the importance of minerals in food is so new that the textbooks on nutritional dietetics contain very little about it. Nevertheless it is something that concerns all of us, and the further we delve into it the more startling it becomes.

You'd think, wouldn't you, that a carrot is a carrot–that one is about as good as another as far as nourishment is concerned? But it isn't; one carrot may look and taste like another and yet be lacking in the particular mineral element which our system requires and which carrots are supposed to contain. Laboratory tests prove that the fruits, the vegetables, the grains, the eggs and even the milk and the meats of today are not what they were a few generations ago. (Which doubtless explains why our forefathers [and foremothers] thrived on a selection of foods that would starve us!) No one of today can eat enough fruits and vegetables to supply their system with the mineral salts they require for perfect health, because their stomach isn't big enough to hold them! And we are running to big stomachs.

No longer does a balanced and fully nourishing diet consist merely of so many calories or certain vitamins or a fixed proportion of starches, proteins, and carbohydrates. We now know that it must contain, in addition, something like a score of mineral salts.

It is bad news to learn from our leading authorities that 99 percent of the American people are deficient in these minerals, and that a marked deficiency in any one of the more important minerals actually results in disease. Any upset of the balance, any considerable lack of one or another element, however microscopic the body requirement may be, and we sicken, suffer, shorten our lives.

This discovery is one of the latest and most important contributions of science to the problem of human health.

So far as the records go, the first man in this field of research, the first to demonstrate that most human foods of our day are poor in minerals and that their proportions are not balanced, was Dr. Charles Northen an Alabama physician now living in Orlando, Florida. His discoveries and achievements are of enormous importance to mankind.

Following a wide experience in general practice, Dr. Northen specialized in stomach diseases and nutritional disorder. Later, he moved to New York and made extensive studies along this line, in conjunction with a famous French scientist from Sorbonne. In the course of that work he convinced himself that there was little authentic, definite information on the chemistry of foods, and that no dependence could be placed on existing data.

He asked himself how foods could be used intelligently in the treatment of disease, when they differed so widely in content. The answer seemed to be that they could not be used intelligently. In

---
200

establishing the fact that serious deficiencies existed and in searching out the reasons therefor, he made an extensive study of the soil. It was he who first voiced the surprising assertion that we must make soil building the basis of food building in order to accomplish human building.

"Bear in mind," says Dr. Northen, "that minerals are vital to human metabolism and health—and that no plant or animal can appropriate to itself any mineral which is not present in the soil upon which it feeds.

"When I first made this statement I was ridiculed, for up to that time people had paid little attention to food deficiencies and even less to soil deficiencies. Men eminent in medicine denied there was any such thing as vegetables and fruits that did not contain sufficient minerals for human needs. Eminent agricultural authorities insisted that all soil contained all necessary minerals. They reasoned that plants take what they need, and that it is the function of the human body to appropriate what it requires. Failure to do so, they said, was a symptom of disorder.

"Some of our respected authorities even claimed that the so-called secondary minerals played no part whatever in human health. It is only recently that such men as Dr. McCollum of Johns Hopkins, Dr. Mendel of Yale, Dr. Sherman of Columbia, Dr. Lipman of Rutgers, and Drs. H.G. Knight and Oswald Schreiner of the United States Department of Agriculture have agreed that these minerals are essential to plant, animal, and human feeding.

"We know that vitamins are complex substances which are indispensable to nutrition, and that each of them is of importance for the normal function of some special structure in the body. Disorder and disease result from any vitamin deficiency.

"It is not commonly realized, however, that vitamins control the body's appropriation of minerals, and in the absence of minerals they have no function to perform. Lacking vitamins, the system can make some use of minerals, but lacking minerals, vitamins are useless.

"Neither does the layman realize that there may be a pronounced difference in both foods and soils—to them one vegetable, one glass of milk, or one egg is about the same as another. Dirt is dirt, too, and they assume that by adding a little fertilizer to it, a satisfactory vegetable or fruit can be grown.

"The truth is that our foods vary enormously in value, and some of them aren't worth eating, as food. For example, vegetation grown in one part of the country may assay 1,100 parts, per billion, of iodine, as against 20 in that grown elsewhere. Processed milk has run anywhere from 362 parts, per million, of iodine and 127 of iron, down to nothing.

"Some of or lands, even unhappily for us, we have been systematically robbing the poor soils and the good soils alike of the very substances most necessary to health, growth, long life, and resistance to disease. Up to the time I began experimenting, almost nothing had been done to make good the theft.

"The more I studied nutritional problems and the effects of mineral deficiencies upon disease, the more plainly I saw that here lay the most direct approach to better health, and the more important it became in my mind to find a method of restoring those missing minerals to our foods.

"The subject interested me so profoundly that I retired from active medical practice and for a good many years now I have devoted myself to it. It's a fascinating subject, for it goes to the heart of human betterment."

The results obtained by Dr. Northen are outstanding. By putting back into foods the stuff that foods are made of, he has proved himself to be a real miracle man of medicine, for he has opened up the shortest and most rational route to better health.

He showed first that it should be done, and then that it could be done. He doubled and redoubled the natural mineral content of fruits and vegetables. He improved the quality of milk by increasing the iron and the iodine in it. He caused hens to lay eggs richer in the vital elements.

By scientific soil feeding, he raised better seed potatoes in Maine, better grapes in California, Better oranges in Florida, and better field crops in other States. (By "better" is meant not only an improvement in food value but also an increase in quantity and quality.)

Before going further into the results he has obtained, let's see just what is involved in this matter of "mineral deficiencies", what it may mean to our health, and how it may effect the growth and development, both mental and physical, of our children.

We know that rats, guinea pigs, and other animals can be fed into a diseased condition and out again by controlling only the minerals in their food.

A 10-year test with rats proved that by withholding calcium they can be bred down to a third the size of those fed with an adequate amount of that mineral. Their intelligence, too, can be controlled by mineral feeding as readily as can their size, their bony structure, and their general health.

Place a number of these little animals inside a maze after starving some of them in a certain mineral element. The starved ones will be unable to find their way out, whereas the others will have little or no difficulty in getting out. Their dispositions can be altered by mineral feeding. They can be made quarrelsome and belligerent; they can even be turned into cannibals and be made to devour each other.

A cage full of normal rats will live in amity. Restrict their calcium, and they will become irritable and draw apart from one another. Then they will begin to fight. Restore their calcium balance and they will grow more friendly; in time they will begin to sleep in a pile as before.

Many backward children are "stupid" merely because they are deficient in magnesia. We punish them for OUR failure to feed them properly.

Certainly our physical well-being is more directly dependent upon the minerals we take into our systems than upon the calories or vitamins or upon the precise proportions of starch, protein, or carbohydrates we consume.

It is now agreed that at least 16 mineral elements are indispensable for normal nutrition, and several more are always found in small amounts in the body, although their precise physiological role has not been determined. Of the 11 indispensable salts, calcium, phosphorous, and iron are perhaps the most important.

Calcium is the dominant nerve controller; it powerfully affects the cell formation of all living things and regulates nerve action. It governs contractability of the muscles and the rhythmic beat of the heart. It also coordinates the other mineral elements and corrects disturbances made by them. It works only in sunlight. Vitamin D is its buddy.

203

Dr. Sherman of Columbia asserts that 50 percent of the American people are starving for calcium. A recent article in the Journal of the American Medical Association stated that out of 4,000 cases in New York Hospital, only 2 were not suffering from a lack of calcium.

What does such a deficiency mean? How would it affect your health or mine? So many morbid conditions and actual diseases may result that it is almost hopeless to catalog them. Included in the list are rickets, bony deformities, bad teeth, nervous disorders, reduced resistance to other diseases, fatigability, and behavior disturbances such as incorrigibility, assaultiveness, nonadaptability.

Here's one specific example: The soil around a certain Midwest city is poor in calcium. Three hundred children of this community were examined and nearly 90 percent and bad teeth, 69 percent showed affections of the nose and throat, swollen glands, enlarged or diseased tonsils. More than one-third had defective vision, round shoulders, bow legs, and anemia.

Calcium and phosphorous appear to pull in double harness. A child requires as much per day as two grown men, but studies indicate a common deficiency of both in our food. Researches on farm animals point to a deficiency of one or the other as the cause of serious losses to the farmers, and when the soil is poor in phosphorous these animals become bone-chewers. Dr. McCollum says that when there are enough phosphates in the blood there can be no dental decay.

Iron is an essential constituent of the oxygen-carrying pigment of the blood: iron starvation results in anemia, and yet iron cannot be assimilated unless some copper is contained in the diet. In Florida many cattle die from an obscure disease called "salt sickness." It has been found to arise from a lack of iron and copper in the soil and hence in the grass. A man may starve for want of these elements just as a beef "critter" starves.

If Iodine is not present in our foods the function of the thyroid gland is disturbed and goiter afflicts us. The human body requires only fourteen-thousandths of a milligram daily, yet we have a distinct "goiter belt" in the Great Lakes section, and in parts of the Northwest the soil is so poor in iodine that the disease is common.

So it goes, down through the list, each mineral element playing a definite role in nutrition. A characteristic set of symptoms, just as specific as any vitamin-deficiency disease, follows a deficiency in any one of them. It is alarming, therefore, to face the fact that we are starving for these precious, health-giving substances.

Very well, you say, if our foods are poor in the mineral salts they are supposed to contain, why not resort to dosing?

That is precisely what is being done, or attempted. However, those who should know assert that the human system cannot appropriate those elements to the best advantage in any but the food form. At best, only a part of them in the form of drugs can be utilized by the body, and certain dieticians go so far as to say it is a waste of effort to fool with them. Calcium, for instance, cannot be supplied in any form of medication with lasting effect.

But there is a more potent reason why the curing of diet deficiencies by drugging hasn't worked out so well. Consider those 16 indispensable elements and those others which presumably perform some obscure function as yet undetermined. Aside from calcium and phosphorous, they are needed only in infinitesimal quantities, and the activity of one may be dependent upon the presence of another. To determine the precise requirements of each individual case and to attempt to weigh it out on a druggist's scale would appear hopeless.

It is a problem and a serious one. But here is the hopeful side of the picture: Nature can and will solve it if she is encouraged to do so. The minerals in fruit and vegetables are colloidal; i.e. they are in a state of such extremely fine suspension that they can be assimilated by the human system: It is merely a question of giving back to nature the materials with which she works.

We must rebuild our soils: Put back the minerals we have taken out. That sounds difficult but it isn't. Neither is it expensive. Therein lies the short cut to better health and longer life.

When Dr. Northen first asserted that many foods were lacking in mineral content and that this deficiency was due solely to an absence of those elements in the soil, his findings were challenged and he was called a crank. But differences of opinion in the medical profession are not uncommon–it was only 60 years ago that the Medical Society of Boston passed a resolution condemning the use of bathtubs — and he persisted in his assertions that inasmuch as foods did not contain what they were supposed to contain, no physician could with certainty prescribe a diet to overcome physical ills.

He showed that the textbooks are not dependable because many of the analyses in them were made many years ago, perhaps from products raised in virgin soils, whereas our soils have been constantly depleted. Soil analysis, he pointed out, reflect only the content of samples. One analysis may be entirely different from another made 10 miles away.

"And so what?" came the query.

Dr. Northen undertook to demonstrate that something could be done about it. By reestablishing a proper soil balance be actually grew crops that contained an ample amount of desired minerals.

This was incredible. It was contrary to the books and it upset everything connected with diet practice. The scoffers began to pay attention to him. Recently the Southern Medical Association, realizing the hopelessness of trying to remedy nutritional deficiencies without positive factors to work with, recommended a careful study to determine the real mineral content of foodstuffs and the variations due to soil depletion in different localities. These progressive medical men are awake to the importance of prevention.

Dr. Northen went even further and proved that crops grown in a properly mineralized soil were bigger and better; that seeds germinated quicker, grew more rapidly and made larger plants; that trees were healthier and put on more fruit of better quality.

By increasing the mineral content of citrus fruit he likewise improved its texture, its appearance and its flavor.

He experimented with a variety of growing things, and in every case the story was the same. By mineralizing the feed at poultry farms, he got more and better eggs; by balancing pasture soils, he produced richer milk. Persistently he hammered home to farmers, to doctors, and to the general public the thought that life depends upon the minerals.

His work led him into a careful study of the effects of climate, sunlight, ultraviolet and thermal rays upon plant, animal, and human hygiene. In consequence he moved to Florida. People familiar with his work consider him the most valuable man in the State. I met him by reason of the fact that I was harassed by certain soil problems on my Florida farm which had baffled the best chemists and fertilizer experts available.

He is an elderly, retiring man, with a warm smile and an engaging personality, He is a trifle shy until he opens up on his pet topic; then his diffidence disappears and he speaks with authority.

His mind is a storehouse crammed with precise, scientific data about soil, and food chemistry, the complicated life processes of plants, animals, and human beings — and the effect of malnutrition upon all three. He is perhaps as close to the secret of life as any man anywhere.

"Do you call yourself a soil or a food chemist?" I inquired.

"Neither. I'm an M.D. My work lies in the field of biochemistry and nutrition. I gave up medicine because this is a wider and more important work. Sick soils mean sick plants, sick animals, and sick people. Physical, mental, and moral fitness depends largely upon an ample supply and a proper proportion of the minerals in our foods. Nerve function, nerve stability, nerve-cell-building likewise depend thereon. I'm really a doctor of sick soils."

"Do you mean to imply that the vegetables I'm raising on my farm are sick?" I asked.

"Precisely! They're as weak and undernourished as anemic children. They're not much good as food. Look at the pests and the disease that plague them. Insecticides cost farmers nearly as much as fertilizers these days.

"A healthy plant, however, grown in soil properly balanced, can and will resist most insect pests. That very characteristic makes it a better food product. You have tuberculosis and pneumonia germ in your system but you're strong enough to throw them off. Similarly, a really healthy plant will pretty nearly take care of itself in the battle against insects and blights –and will also give the human system what it requires."

"Good heavens! Do you realize what that means to agriculture?"

"Perfectly. Enormous saving. Better crops. Lowered living costs to the rest of us. But I'm not so much interested in agriculture as in health."

"It sounds beautifully theoretical and utterly impractical to me," I told the doctor, whereupon he gave me some of his case records.

For instance, in an orange grove infested with scale, when he restored the mineral balance to part of the soil, the trees growing in that part became clean while the rest remained diseased. By the same means he had grown healthy rosebushes between rows that were riddled by insects.

He had grown tomato and cucumber plants, both healthy and diseased, where the vines intertwined. The bugs ate up the diseased and refused to touch the healthy plants! He showed me interesting analysis of citrus fruit, the chemistry and the food value of which accurately reflected the soil treatment the trees had received.

There is no space here to go fully into Dr. Northen's work but it is of such importance as to rank with that of Burbank, the plant wizard, and with that of our famous physiologists and nutritional experts.

"Healthy plants mean healthy people", said he. "We can't raise a strong race on a weak soil. Why don't you try mending the deficiencies on your farm and growing more minerals into your crops?"

I did try and I succeeded. I was planting a large acreage of celery and under Dr. Northen's direction I fed minerals into certain blocks of the land in varying amounts. When the plants from this soil were mature I had them analyzed, along with celery from other parts of the State. It was the most careful and comprehensive study of the kind ever made, and it included over 250 separate chemical determinations. I was amazed to learn that my celery had more than twice the mineral content of the best grown elsewhere. Furthermore, it kept much better, with and without refrigeration, proving that the cell structure was sounder.

In 1927, Mr. W. W. Kincaid, a "gentleman farmer" of Niagara Falls, heard an address by Dr. Northen and was so impressed that he began extensive experiments in the mineral feeding of plants and animals. The results he has accomplished are conspicuous. He set himself the task of increasing the iodine in the milk from his dairy herd. He has succeeded in adding both iodine and iron so liberally that one glass of his milk contains all of these minerals that an adult person requires for a day.

Is this significant? Listen to these incredible figures taken from a bulletin of the South Carolina Food Research Commission: "In many sections three out of five persons have goiter and a recent estimate states that 30 million people in the United States suffer from it."

Foods rich in iodine are of the greatest importance to these sufferers.

Mr Kincaid took a brown Swiss heifer calf which was dropped in the stockyards, and by raising her on mineralized pasturage and a properly balanced diet made her the third all-time champion of her breed! In one season she gave 21,924 pounds of milk. He raised her butterfat production from 410 pounds in 1 year to 1,037 pounds. Results like these are of incalculable importance.

Others besides Mr. Kincaid are following the trail Dr. Northen blazed. Similar experiments with milk have been made in Illinois and nearly every fertilizer company is beginning to urge use of the rare mineral elements. As an example I quote from statements of a subsidiary of one of the leading copper companies:

Many States show a marked reduction in the productive capacity of the soil * * * in many districts amounting to a 25 to 50 percent reduction in the last 50 years * * *. Some areas show a tenfold variation in calcium. Some show a sixtyfold variation in phosphorus * * *. Authorities * * * see soil depletion, barren livestock, increased human death rate due to heart disease, deformities, arthritis, increased dental caries, all due to lack of essential minerals in plant food.

"It is neither a complicated nor an expensive undertaking to restore our soils to balance and thereby work a real miracle in the control of disease," says Dr. Northen. "As a matter of fact, it's a money-making move for the farmer, and any competent soil chemist can tell them how to proceed.

"First determine by analysis the precise chemistry of any given soil, then correct the deficiencies by putting down enough of the missing elements to restore its balance. The same care should be used as in prescribing for a sick patient, for proportions are of vital importance.

"In my early experiments I found it extremely difficult to get the variety of minerals needed in the form in which I wanted to use them but advancement in chemistry, and especially our ever-increasing knowledge of colloidal chemistry, has solved that difficulty. It is now possible, by use of minerals in colloidal form, to prescribe a cheap and effective system of soil correction which meets this vital need and one which fits in admirably with nature's plans.

"Soils seriously deficient in minerals cannot produce plant life competent to maintain our needs, and with the continuous cropping and shipping away of those concentrates, the condition becomes worse.

"A famous nutrition authority recently said, 'One sure way to end the American people's susceptibility to infection is to supply through food a balanced ration of iron, copper, and other metals. An organism supplied with a diet adequate to, or preferably in excess of, all mineral requirements may so utilize these elements as to produce artificially by our present method of immunization. You can't make up the deficiency by using patent medicine.'

"He's absolutely right. Prevention of disease is easier, more practical, and more economical than cure, but not until foods are standardized on a basis of what they contain instead of what they look like can the dietician prescribe them with intelligence and with effect.

"There was a time when medical therapy had no standards because the therapeutic elements in drugs had not been definitely determined on a chemical basis. Pharmaceutical houses have changed all that. Food chemistry, on the other hand, has depended almost entirely upon governmental agencies for its research, and in our real knowledge of values we are about where medicine was a century ago.

"Disease preys most surely and most viciously on the undernourishment and unfit plants, animals, and human beings alike, and when the importance of these obscure mineral elements is fully realized the chemistry of life will have to be rewritten. No one knows their mental or bodily capacity, how well they can feel or how long they can live, for we are all cripples and weaklings. It is a disgrace to science. Happily, that chemistry is being rewritten and we are on our way to better health by returning to the soil the things we have stolen from it.

"The public can help; it can hasten the change. How? By demanding quality in its food. By insisting that our doctors and our health departments establish scientific standards of nutritional value.

"The growers will quickly respond. They can put back those minerals almost overnight, and by doing so they can actually make money through bigger and better crops.

"It is simpler to cure sick soils than sick people — which shall we choose?"

www.betterhealththruresearch.com/US SenateDocument.htm
bioelectrichelth.org/MMM 1936.htm

About the Author

Dr. Kelly Miller is a 1980 graduate of Logan University of Health Sciences in St. Louis, Missouri, receiving his Doctor of Chiropractic degree.

He received a Certification in Industrial/Occupational Health from Northwestern Chiropractic College in 1991.

He worked as an ergonomic, safety-consultant and after-care doctor for Food Barn, Ball's Price Chopper, and Twentieth Century in the Kansas City Metropolitan area in the 1990's.

He received his certificate in Acupuncture in 1996, and is a Fellow of the Acupuncture Society of America.

In 2001, he received his Certification as a Naturopathic Medical Doctor from the National Accreditation and Certification of Naturopathic Medical Doctors in Washington DC.

He finished his Fellowship in Aging and Regenerative Medicine from the Brazil-American Academy of Aging and Regenerative Medicine in San Paulo, Brazil, in March 2014.

He received his Certification in Functional Diagnostic Medicine from Functional Medicine University in December 2014.

Dr. Miller's clinical practice covers over thirty-five years, treating over fifteen thousand patients. He is an international lecturer on the genetic, nutritional, and hormonal considerations related to heart health.

The following is an excerpt from Dr. Miller's next book, *Micronutrient Testing: How To Find What Nutrients Your Body Needs.*

I discovered the importance of nutrition in 1978 at the age of twenty-two when my senior clinician at chiropractic school recommended I stop drinking milk and start taking betaine HCL with my meals. I was amazed and pleasantly surprised to find my digestive dysfunction and reoccurring urinary tract infections went away and never returned. One of my early mentors was Dr. MT Morter, Jr., who was president of Logan University while I attended and later authored several books. He was a proponent of alkalizing the body with foods and supplements that contained potassium, magnesium, zinc, selenium, and the like. One of the supplements I recommended in those days for my patients was *Green Magma*, a green powder made from barley sprouts because of its mineral content. Generally speaking, the patient population of the late seventies and early eighties were a much healthier lot than the patients of today.

It has been known for some time that there have been significant mineral and vitamin deficiencies in the soil and the food sources in the United States for over eighty years. I found an interesting article from *Cosmopolitan* magazine concerning a report from Congress in 1936 about this mineral loss in the soil and foods in the U.S. (See this article in the Appendix.) Things have not gotten better since 1936, but are worse, much worse. It is not a question if you have a nutritional deficiency, you do. It is more of a question of how many are there and how severe are they?

Today, we have the technology to evaluate specific vitamin, mineral, amino acids, fatty acids, and anti-oxidants in individuals. There is no more guesswork in determining the specific nutritional needs of any individual.

I hope you enjoy the book. God Bless.
Kelly Miller DC NMD FASA FBAARM CFMP